Calm Your Anger Now

Stop Your Rage, Ease Anxiety,
Lower Stress, and Learn to
Control Your Emotions in
Everyday Life

Alex M. Langston

professional before attempting any techniques outlined in this book.

By reading this document, the reader agrees that under no circumstances is the author responsible for any losses, direct or indirect, that are incurred as a result of the use of the information contained within this document, including, but not limited to, errors, omissions, or inaccuracies.

Table of Contents

INTRODUCTION 1

CHAPTER 1: STRESSES IN TODAY'S WORLD 3

WHAT IS ANGER? 3

EMOTIONAL RESPONSE TO ANGER 4

WHY DO WE EXPERIENCE ANGER? 4

THE IMPACT OF ANGER 5

THREE STAGES OF ANGER 5

CONSTRUCTIVE ANGER 6

DESTRUCTIVE ANGER 7

SYMPATHETIC NERVOUS SYSTEM AND ANGER 7

PARASYMPATHETIC NERVOUS SYSTEM AND ANGER 8

CAUSES OF ANGER 9

FINANCIAL PROBLEMS 10

WORK-RELATED STRESS 10

RELATIONSHIP PROBLEMS 10

HEALTH CONCERNS 11

FAMILY CONCERNS 11

PARENTING 11

TIME MANAGEMENT 12

DAILY LIFE AND BUSYNESS 12

EIGHT MODERN LIFE STRESSORS 12

NINE ANTIDOTES FOR MODERN LIFE STRESSORS 14

FIVE MYTHS ABOUT ANGER 15

CHAPTER 2: EFFECTS OF ANGER AND STRESS 17

LONG-TERM HEALTH EFFECTS 17

NEGATIVE SOCIAL EFFECTS 17

INCREASED LEVEL OF HOSTILITY 18

INCREASED JOB STRESS 18

FAMILY CONFLICT 18

DEPRESSION 18

COMMON EFFECTS OF STRESS 19

EFFECTS ON YOUR BODY 19

SLEEP PROBLEMS 20

CHANGE IN SEX DRIVE 20

OVER OR UNDER-EATING 21

LESS PHYSICAL ACTIVITY 21

DRUG OR ALCOHOL ABUSE 21

TOBACCO USE 22

EFFECTS ON YOUR MOOD 22

ANXIETY 22

IRRITABILITY 22

RESTLESSNESS 23

ANGRY OUTBURSTS 23

LACK OF MOTIVATION OR FOCUS 23

FEELING OVERWHELMED 23

CHAPTER 3: IS YOUR LIFESTYLE TO BLAME? 25

HOW DO YOU EXPRESS YOURSELF RIGHT NOW? 26
HOW DID YOU LEARN TO EXPRESS YOURSELF? 27
WHAT IS YOUR SOCIAL CIRCLE LIKE NOW? 28
DO YOU HAVE ANY SUPPORT SYSTEMS IN PLACE? 28

CHAPTER 4: THE DIFFERENT EMOTIONS AT PLAY 29

PRIMARY AND SECONDARY EMOTIONS 29
THE DIFFERENT TYPES OF ANGER 29

ANGER AND ITS OTHER EMOTIONS 32
DISPLACED ANGER 35

CHAPTER 5: UNDERSTANDING YOUR
TRIGGERS 37

WHAT ARE TRIGGERS? 37
TYPES OF TRIGGERS 38
WHO ARE YOU? 38
HOW TO HANDLE TRIGGERS 39
WHAT NOT TO DO 40
WHAT ARE SOME COMMON TRIGGERS? 41
AVOID PROVOCATIONS 42
FIND SOLUTIONS TO SOCIAL PROBLEMS42

STYLES OF SOCIAL PROBLEM-SOLVING 43

STEPS OF SOCIAL PROBLEM-SOLVING 44

CHAPTER 6: UNDERSTANDING YOUR END
GOAL 47

WHY ARE YOU ANGRY? 47
PINPOINT THE GOAL OF YOUR
ANGER 48
WHAT IS YOUR ANGER TRYING TO TELL
YOU? 49
THE ROOT OF ANGER 49
THERAPIES AND UNDERSTANDING
YOUR ANGER 50

CHAPTER 7: BALANCING YOUR LIFE 53

CAUSES OF AN UNBALANCED LIFE 53

SIGNS THAT YOU MAY HAVE AN UNBALANCED LIFE 57
CONTROLLING ANGER EQUALS FINDING THE BALANCE BETWEEN SNS AND PNS 58
COUNTERBALANCING STRESS TO IMPROVE OUR HEALTH 59

START WITH YOURSELF FIRST 60

MAKE TIME FOR THE THINGS YOU LOVE 61

CHECK YOUR THOUGHTS 61

GET OUTSIDE AND STEP OUT OF YOUR MIND 62

CHOOSE YOUR BATTLES 62

BE PROACTIVE 62

BE PRESENT 63

MAKE TIME FOR YOURSELF 63

CHAPTER 8: WAYS OF COPING WITH AND CONTROLLING ANGER 65

DISTRESS TOLERANCE—DBT SKILLS 65
PRACTICING RADICAL ACCEPTANCE 68
IN THE MOMENT COOL DOWN TECHNIQUES 69

LEAVE THE SITUATION 69

CHANGE YOUR THOUGHTS 70

RELAXATION TECHNIQUES AND MEDITATION 70

CONVINCE YOURSELF TO CALM DOWN 71

USE HUMOR 71

RESOLVING CONFLICT 72

EXPRESS YOUR EMOTIONS EFFECTIVELY 72

PRACTICE ACTIVE LISTENING SKILLS 72

NEGOTIATE OR COMPROMISE WHEN NECESSARY 73

USE DEAR MAN 73

OTHER HELPFUL TECHNIQUES 74

RECOGNIZE THE WARNING SIGNS 74

UNDERSTAND YOUR ANGER 75

WRITE IT OUT 75

COUNT TO 100 76

PRESS PAUSE 76

MOVE AROUND 76

TALK TO SOMEONE 76

TAKE TIME FOR YOURSELF 77

BIOFEEDBACK 77

MEDITATION 77

MINDFULNESS 78

CHAPTER 9: ANGER KILLS! MANAGE YOUR
ANGER 79

RESPONSES TO ANGER 79

FOUR PRIMARY WAYS OF EXPRESSING
AGGRESSION OR ANGER 79

HOW TO UNDERSTAND YOUR ANGER ... 80
EMOTION REGULATION—DBT SKILLS .. 82

CHANGING THE WAY YOU RESPOND TO YOUR
ANGER 82

WAYS TO HANDLE YOUR ANGER 84
10 "QUICK FIXES" FOR ANGER
MANAGEMENT 87
OTHER ANGER MANAGEMENT
TOOLS 90

COPING WITH STRESS 92

CHAPTER 10: IMPROVE YOUR SOCIAL AND
INTERPERSONAL SKILLS 97

INTERPERSONAL EFFECTIVENESS—DBT
SKILLS 97

WHAT ARE INTERPERSONAL EFFECTIVENESS
SKILLS? 97

WHY ARE INTERPERSONAL EFFECTIVENESS SKILLS IMPORTANT? 98

WHAT ARE SOME TIPS FOR USING INTERPERSONAL EFFECTIVENESS SKILLS? 98

BE AWARE OF YOUR BODY LANGUAGE . 99
ELEMENTS OF BODY LANGUAGE 100

EYE CONTACT 100

FACIAL EXPRESSIONS 101

GESTURES 101

POSTURE 101

INTERPERSONAL SPACE 101

TONE OF VOICE 102

BE AN ACTIVE LISTENER 102
AREAS OF INTERPERSONAL SKILLS 103

COMMUNICATION SKILLS 103

MANAGING DIFFERENCES 104

CREATE A HARMONIOUS TEAM 105

PERSONAL INTEGRITY 106

GIVE ACRONYM 107
FAST ACRONYM 107
THINK ACRONYM 108
BOUNDARY BUILDING SKILLS 109

WHAT ARE BOUNDARY BUILDING SKILLS? .. 109

WHY ARE BOUNDARY BUILDING SKILLS
IMPORTANT?.. 109

HOW CAN I IMPROVE MY BOUNDARY
BUILDING SKILLS? 109

CHAPTER 11: RESILIENCE AND
RESOLUTION—BUILDING STRENGTH......113

WHAT IS RESILIENCE? 113
HOW CAN I BUILD RESILIENCE? 113
DEVELOPING A GROWTH MINDSET 115

HOW TO DEVELOP A GROWTH MINDSET 116

SIX STEPS TO BUILD RESILIENCE 117

NOTICE YOUR STRESS RESPONSES 117

LEAVE YOUR MIND AND TURN TO THE
PRESENT MOMENT 118

HEALTHY HABITS ARE A PRIORITY 118

FIND MEANING AND CONNECT WITH YOUR
TASKS 119

EMPATHY, EMPATHY, AND MORE
EMPATHY 119

YOU ARE THE DRIVER OF YOUR LIFE 119

SEVEN C'S OF RESILIENCE: A FORMULA
FOR SUCCESS 120

CHAPTER 12: CULTIVATING THE RIGHT ATTITUDE AND CREATING AN ACTION PLAN 123

HOW ATTITUDE CAN REDUCE YOUR STRESS LEVELS 123

THOUGHTS ARE THE CREATOR OF EXPERIENCE 124

HOW TO REFRAME YOUR THOUGHTS 124

CREATIVE WAYS TO KEEP A POSITIVE ATTITUDE 125

ADDITIONAL TACTICS FOR A POSITIVE MIND 126

HOW TO GET RID OF STRESS 127

CREATING YOUR ACTION PLAN 128

ACTION PLAN TEMPLATE 130

CONCLUSION 135

REFERENCES 137

Introduction

How would you describe yourself? Do you get angry easily? Do you get impatient often? Are you susceptible to violent outbursts or have a "short fuse?" Does your family often describe their interactions with you as having to "walk on eggshells" or "walking on thin ice?" If you've answered yes to any of these questions, then this book is for you! Choosing this book likely means you're looking for ways to improve your anger management skills, ease your anxiety, and be more in control of your emotions in everyday life. The help you need is right here in this book.

Anger is a powerful emotion. Everyone experiences it from time to time, but it's difficult to deal with. Anger can boil within us until it eventually combusts unhealthily. However, it can also manifest into different emotions or physical responses. It can be a loud and aggressive outburst or it can be a subtle feeling of annoyance or frustration. No matter how it's expressed, anger is often seen as a negative emotion. We're taught from a young age that it's bad to get angry; that we should always try to stay calm.

What if we told you that anger isn't always a bad thing? Anger can actually be beneficial! It can be a motivator; a way to push yourself to do better. It can also be a sign that something is wrong and needs to be changed. Anger is a natural emotion, and it's okay to feel angry. The goal isn't to eliminate anger, but to learn how to deal with it healthily. Otherwise, it can damage our relationships, careers, and even our physical health if we don't know how to deal with it properly.

If you're struggling to control your anger, don't worry—many others are in a similar boat. Luckily, anger is a manageable emotion. With the right techniques, you can learn how to control it and lead a healthier, happier life. This guide will take you through the basics of anger management so that you can take control of your emotions and live a calmer, more peaceful life. In this book, you'll learn:

- how to identify the signs that you need anger management,
- how to understand the various forms of anger,
- how to find healthy ways to express your anger,
- how to develop a plan to manage your anger,
- and much more!

By the end of this book, you'll have all the tools you need to manage your anger in a healthy way. If you're ready to learn how to calm your anger and take back control of your life, then let's get started! Don't let your stress and anger take control—take control of your anger and start living a calmer, happier life today!

Chapter 1:

Stresses in Today's World

The 21st century is a stressful time to be alive. With the world becoming more and more connected, we're constantly bombarded with new information and demands on our time. From work to families to social media, it's easy to feel overwhelmed and like you can't keep up.

And that's before we even get to the big stuff: climate change, political instability, and economic uncertainty. It's no wonder that so many of us are feeling stressed out!

But don't despair—you can manage your stress and live a happier, healthier life. In this chapter, we'll explore some of the most common causes of stress and how to deal with them.

What Is Anger?

Anger is an emotion that is characterized by feelings of frustration, hostility, and aggression. Anger can be triggered or caused by a variety of challenges, including stress, annoyance, and fear. When you get angry, you might notice that your heart rate increases, your muscles tense up, and you might breathe faster. Anger can influence the *fight-or-flight* (sometimes called the *fight-flight-or-freeze*) response in your body.

Emotional Response to Anger

The emotional response to anger can vary from person to person. Some people might feel like they're about to explode, while others might just feel mildly annoyed. It's important to understand your own emotional response to anger so that you can deal with it healthily. When we're angry, we might feel like we want to scream and blow up at whoever wronged us. We might also feel like our heart is racing, our muscles are tense, and we're breathing more quickly. We might feel like we need to scream or hit something. Anger can elicit a sense of panic or anxiety in some people.

Why Do We Experience Anger?

There are several reasons behind experiencing anger. Sometimes, anger can be caused by stress or frustration. Maybe you're feeling overwhelmed by your workload or you're dealing with a difficult situation at home. Or maybe you're just feeling generally stressed and angry about the state of the world. In other cases, anger might be caused by annoyance or irritation.

Maybe someone cut you off in traffic or your co-worker keeps stealing your lunch from the fridge. Or maybe you're just sick and tired of dealing with a particular problem and you're ready to lash out. Or perhaps you've calmly asked your child eight times to tidy their room or what they want for dinner, only to be ignored. Occasionally, anger might be caused by fear. Maybe you're afraid of something that's happening in your life or in the world. Or maybe you're feeling threatened or helpless in a situation.

In general, anger is a normal and even helpful response to certain situations. It can prompt us to challenge stress and motivate us to take action. However, when anger interferes with our daily lives, it might be time to get some help.

The Impact of Anger

Anger can impact our lives in several ways. In some cases, it might lead to problems at work or in our relationships. It can also impact our physical health, leading to issues with high blood pressure or heart disease. If we don't manage our anger appropriately, it can lead to destructive behaviors like substance abuse or violence.

Three Stages of Anger

There are three stages of anger. The first stage is when you feel the **initial anger**. This is the fight-or-flight response. As stated before, this response incorporates the release of adrenaline and cortisol. It's meant to protect you from danger and help you escape or fight the threat. This response is instinctual and happens automatically.

The second stage is **resistance**. This occurs when your body attempts to return to homeostasis. Your heart rate and blood pressure decrease, and you might notice that your muscles start to relax. This is the stage where you might feel calmer. However, if your body doesn't return to homeostasis, you might enter the third stage of anger.

The third stage is **exhaustion**. This is when your body has used up all its resources to cope with the stressor. You might feel tired, both physically and mentally. This is the stage where you're more likely to make impulsive decisions or act out in anger. It's important to note that not everyone experiences all three stages of anger. And people can move through the stages at different speeds. For example, some people might go from feeling angry to feeling calm within a matter of minutes. Others might take hours or days to calm down.

Constructive Anger

It's important to understand that not all anger is bad. In fact, anger can be a constructive emotion. It can motivate you to take action or change your life. For example, if you're angry about the state of the world, you might be motivated to get involved in politics or volunteer for a cause you care about. If you're angry about a situation at work, you might gain the courage to speak up or make changes in your workplace.

If you're angry about a problem in your personal life, you might be motivated to change your relationships or your lifestyle. Anger can also be a helpful emotion in the moment. It can give you the energy and motivation you need to get through a difficult situation. Remember, anger is a part of the natural fight-or-flight response. It's designed to help us survive and cope with stress.

While anger can be constructive, it can also be destructive. When anger is destructive, it leads to problems in our lives and relationships. It can also cause health problems. Destructive anger is often the result of unresolved conflict or unaddressed problems. When we bottle up our anger or try to suppress it, it can lead to problems down the road. It's important to find healthy ways to deal with our anger. This might include talking to a therapist, journaling, or practicing meditation or mindfulness.

Sympathetic Nervous System and Anger

The sympathetic nervous system (SNS) monitors the fight-or-flight response. This is the automatic response that occurs when we feel threatened. The SNS triggers the release of adrenaline and cortisol. These hormones prepare the body to take action against a threat. They increase heart rate, blood pressure, and respiration. They also decrease blood flow to the digestive system and increase blood flow to the muscles. This response protects us from danger and helps us escape or fight the threat. During this stage, you might experience emotional, behavioral, interpersonal, and physical symptoms.

- **Behavioral symptoms**: clenched fists, grinding teeth, outbursts, or pacing
- **Interpersonal symptoms**: feeling like you need to protect yourself or others

- **Physical symptoms**: increased heart rate, sweating, and tension in the muscles
- **Emotional symptoms**: a feeling of anger, anxiety, or fear

Parasympathetic Nervous System and Anger

The parasympathetic nervous system (PNS) handles the *rest-and-digest* response. This is the response that occurs when we're at rest or doing activities that don't require a lot of energy. The PNS triggers the release of hormones that help the body relax and promote a sense of calm. These hormones include serotonin and oxytocin. The PNS:

- promotes relaxation
- lowers heart rate
- decreases blood pressure
- slows respiration
- increases blood flow to the digestive system

The benefits of the PNS are:

- relaxation
- lower stress levels
- reduced anxiety
- improved mood
- better sleep
- increased concentration

Causes of Anger

Anger can arise for a number of reasons. Some causes are external, like another person's actions or a stressful event. Other causes are internal, like our thoughts or emotions. And sometimes, it can be a combination of both.

External causes are:

- **Other people's actions**. If someone cuts you off in traffic, doesn't hold the door open for you, a person is generally rude, kids not listening, or hurting their siblings can trigger anger.

- **Stressful events**. If you're going through a tough time at work or in your personal life, it can lead to anger.

Internal causes are:

- **Thoughts**. If you're constantly thinking negative thoughts, it can lead to anger. For example, if you tell yourself that you're not good enough or that someone is out to get you, it can make you angry.

- **Emotions**. If you're feeling sad, frustrated, or anxious, it can lead to anger.

Anger can be triggered by common, everyday problems like the following.

Financial Problems

For many of us, money is a major source of stress. Whether we're worried about bills, trying to save for a big purchase, or dealing with debt, financial problems can leave a mark on our mental and physical health. Especially after the unpredictability that remained in the wake of the COVID-19 pandemic, we're left worrying about our financial stability more than ever.

Work-Related Stress

For most of us, work is a necessary part of life. However, it can also be a major source of stress. Whether we're worried about job security, dealing with difficult co-workers, or simply feeling overwhelmed by our workload, work-related stress is a common problem. The pandemic has only made things worse, with many of us working from home in less than ideal conditions but are fighting to discover that perfect work-life balance.

Relationship Problems

Our relationships with family, friends, and romantic partners can be a major source of joy—but they can also be another primary source of stress. Conflict, communication problems, and different lifestyles can all put a strain on even the strongest relationships. And when things are going wrong, it's hard to feel like anything else in your life is going right.

Health Concerns

Our physical health is also a common source of stress. Whether we're dealing with a chronic illness, coping with an injury, or simply trying to stay healthy as we age, our physical health can have a big impact on our stress levels. And when we're worried about our health, it's hard to focus on anything else.

Family Concerns

Our families can be a substantial source of support—but they can also add to our daily stressors. Whether we're dealing with difficult family dynamics, caring for aging parents, or worrying about our children, family stress is a common problem. With families struggling to transition to virtual schooling and working from home, this stress is more prevalent now than ever.

Parenting

For parents, stress is often unavoidable. Whether we're dealing with tantrums, sleep problems, or simply the day-to-day challenges of caring for a child, parenting stress can be a big part of our lives. And as our children get older and we face new challenges, like teenage rebellion or college costs, the stress can only increase. While parenting is a wonderful part of life, filled with joy and love, it's also normal to feel overwhelmed at times.

Time Management

In our fast-paced world, it's easy to feel like we're always running behind. With so much to do and so little time to do it, it's no wonder that time management is a major source of stress for many of us. If you're always feeling like you're playing catch-up, it's time to reassess your priorities by changing your viewpoint. By learning to manage your time more effectively, you can reduce your stress levels and enjoy a more relaxed lifestyle.

Daily Life and Busyness

The hustle and bustle of daily life can be a major source of stress. Whether we're dealing with traffic, fighting crowds, or simply trying to get through our never-ending to-do lists, the busyness of life can affect our mental and physical health. If you're feeling overwhelmed by the pace of life, take a step back and focus on what's really important.

Eight Modern Life Stressors

1. **Always on**. We're never off; we're always connected. With technology, we're always reachable and always on. We feel the need to be constantly involved while juggling work, family, and social obligations.

2. **Bombarded**. We're constantly bombarded with stimuli. From 24-hour news cycles to social media, we're constantly inundated with

information and stimuli, which can make us feel overwhelmed.

3. **Go, go, go**! We're always on the go. Our fast-paced way of living leaves little time for rest and relaxation. We're constantly on the go, and this can lead to feelings of being overwhelmed and stressed.

4. **Decisions, decisions**. We're constantly overwhelmed by choices. From what to wear, to what to eat, to where to live—we're constantly facing choices, which can lead to stress.

5. **Blurred priorities**. With so much going on, it's difficult to prioritize and focus on what's important. When we can't prioritize, we can feel anxious and overwhelmed with an endless list of tasks to accomplish.

6. **Can't cope**. When we don't have healthy coping mechanisms in place, we're more likely to feel stressed. This can include things like poor sleep hygiene, an unhealthy diet, and excessive alcohol consumption.

7. **Pollution**. We're constantly surrounded by pollution, both in the air we breathe and the water we drink. This can lead to feelings of anxiety and stress.

8. **Diet**. Fast food, junk food, and alcohol consumption can have negative effects on health and appearance, causing stress or anxiety.

Nine Antidotes for Modern Life Stressors

There's no perfect antidote, but there are some things that can help. Here are a few ideas:

1. **Unplug and disconnect**. Take some time each day to disconnect from technology and the outside world. This can help you relax and recharge.

2. **K.I.S.S. (Keep it simple silly)**. Declutter your home, reduce your possessions, and streamline your schedule. This can help you focus on what's important and reduce stress.

3. **You are enough**. You can't please everyone all the time, and that's okay. Learn to say no to things that don't align with your values or that will add unnecessary stress to your life.

4. **Learn to cope**. Put in the effort to learn coping and relaxation techniques. Yoga, meditation, and reading this book, can all help with dealing with your stress more constructively.

5. **Quality sleep**. Getting the right amount of quality sleep is crucial for managing stress. Make sure you're getting seven to eight hours of sleep each night. However, the quality of sleep is also crucial. Reduce the use of technology in the bedroom, avoid using your phone an hour before bed and an hour before waking, and don't eat or drink before bed.

6. **Exercise regularly**. Exercise releases endorphins, which have mood-boosting effects. This can help you cope with stress healthily.

7. **Nature**. Connecting with nature induces positivity and improves your mood. Get outside for a walk or hike in the park regularly.

8. **Wellbeing**. Increasing your resilience can help you better cope with stress. You can boost your resilience by practicing gratitude, setting realistic goals, and cultivating a positive mindset.

9. **Get creative.** Singing, painting, sketching, dancing, writing, and playing music even for 10 minutes a day has been proven to ease anxiety and stress.

Five Myths About Anger

The myths that pertain to anger can make it tougher to deal with. It's important to understand the truths about anger so that you can manage it in a healthy way.

Myth 1: Anger is always bad.

Anger isn't always bad. In fact, anger can be a healthy emotion. It's only when anger is mismanaged that it becomes a problem.

Myth 2: You should never express anger.

Suppressing anger can actually make it worse. Having healthy outlets to express your anger is crucial.

Instead, talk to a friend, write in a journal, go for a run, paint, draw or play music.

Myth 3: Anger is always caused by someone else.

While other people can certainly trigger our anger, they're not always the root cause. Often, our anger is caused by our own thoughts and beliefs. For example, we might get angry at our boss for being demanding, but the root cause of our anger might be our own perfectionism.

Myth 4: You should never get angry at yourself.

It's perfectly normal to feel anger towards yourself. In fact, self-anger can be a helpful emotion. It can motivate you to change your life or help you deal with past hurts.

Myth 5: Ignoring feelings makes them disappear.

When we try to ignore our anger, it doesn't just go away. In fact, suppressed anger can actually make us physically and mentally ill. Expressing anger appropriately is crucial to its "disappearance."

Anger is a perfectly normal emotion. Poor anger control is the issue. If you're struggling to deal with your anger, there are many resources available to help you. You can talk to a therapist, snuggle with a self-help book (like this one), or join a support group. Remember, you don't have to deal with your anger alone. There are people who can help.

Chapter 2:

Effects of Anger and Stress

Anger and stress are normal human emotions. However, when they're not managed properly, they can lead to concerns. Anger can lead to physical violence, while stress can lead to anxiety and depression.

Long-Term Health Effects

Anger and stress can also impact your physical health. Chronic anger has been linked to high blood pressure, stroke, heart disease, and other health problems. Stress can also weaken your immune system, making you more susceptible to illness.

Negative Social Effects

Anger and stress can also have negative social effects. When you're angry, you're more likely to say or do something you'll regret. This can damage your relationships and make it difficult to connect with others. Stress can also lead to social withdrawal, as you may avoid people and situations that trigger your stress.

Increased Level of Hostility

If you feel angry more often than usual, it could be a sign that your stress levels are too high. Maybe you feel you're constantly on edge, or maybe you're quick to lash out at those around you. Either way, it's important to manage your stress. When stress is left unchecked, it can lead to an increased level of hostility. This can manifest itself as verbal or physical outbursts.

Increased Job Stress

Job stress is a common source of stress for many people. If you're feeling overwhelmed at work, it's important to reduce your stress. Maybe you need to delegate some of your tasks, take a break from work, or communicate better with your boss.

Family Conflict

Family conflict is another common source of stress. If you're constantly arguing with your family, it's important to resolve the conflict. Perhaps you need to set boundaries, communicate better, or spend less time with your family. This can include things like family therapy, mediation, and open communication.

Depression

Depression is a mental health disorder that can be caused by stress. Maybe you're feeling sad, hopeless, or empty. Perhaps you're losing interest in activities you once enjoyed or have trouble sleeping. If you're experiencing these symptoms, it's important to get help. Therapy, medication, and self-care can all be helpful in treating depression.

Common Effects of Stress

There are several common effects of stress, both short-term and long-term. Short-term effects of stress include things like headaches, insomnia, and indigestion. Long-term effects of stress include anxiety, depression, and heart disease.

Effects on Your Body

Your body responds to stress in several ways. Your heart rate and blood pressure increase, you may perspire, and your muscles may tense up. This is our good old friend, the fight-or-flight response, and it's your body's way of preparing you to deal with a stressor.

You may also experience:

- **Headaches**

Migraines and tension and cluster headaches are only a few examples of headaches that can be caused by stress. If you're experiencing headaches, it's important to see a doctor to rule out any other potential causes.

- **Muscle tension or pain**

Muscle tension and pain are the common effects of stress. If you're feeling tense or in pain, it's important to relax your body. Exercise, yoga, and massages can all be helpful in relieving muscle tension.

- **Stomach problems**

Stress can cause a variety of stomach problems, such as indigestion, heartburn, and ulcers. It's also been linked to digestion diseases like Crohn's or irritable bowel syndrome (IBS).

- **Chest pains**

Stress can cause chest pain, which may feel like a heart attack. You may have trouble breathing and your chest feels tight. If you're experiencing chest pains often and are concerned, visit a doctor to have them evaluate your situation.

Sleep Problems

Stress can cause sleep problems, such as insomnia and nightmares. If you're having trouble sleeping, incorporate some relaxing routines before bed. Reading, taking a warm bath, or basking in calm music can all help you get a good night's sleep. Additionally, the blue light that our electronic devices emit emulates the same effects as sunlight, which can interrupt our circadian rhythm, so limit the use of technology before sleeping and after waking.

Change in Sex Drive

Stress can cause either an increase or decrease in your sex drive. Your drive might be a coping mechanism for your stress. Or your drive may lower if you feel poorly about yourself. If you're experiencing a change in your sex drive, it's important to talk to your doctor to rule out other concerns. Sex can also be of great help in relieving stress. When practiced safely and responsibly, the body produces the hormones serotonin and oxytocin, which ease anxiety and stress.

Over or Under-Eating

Stress can lead to over- or under-eating. Changes in your appetite may comprise either not wanting to eat at all or wanting to eat all the time. Your diet might shift toward an interest in unhealthy foods as well. If you're experiencing changes in your appetite, it's important to talk to a doctor or nutritionist to make sure you're getting the nutrients you need.

Less Physical Activity

Less physical activity is a common effect of stress. You may not feel like exercising or you may be too tired to exercise. Or maybe you'd rather spend all day in bed instead of going to work. Taking walks, going to the gym, or doing other types of exercise can help you reduce your stress and redirect your life. If you're experiencing less physical activity, talk to your doctor to see if there's a medical reason for it.

Drug or Alcohol Abuse

Drug or alcohol abuse is common when stressors take over. Drug or alcohol abuse can lead to addiction and other serious health problems. If you're struggling with drug or alcohol abuse, seek help from a professional.

Treatment centers can help you tackle your addiction and get your life back on track.

Tobacco Use

Tobacco use can result from being overwhelmed. It can lead to addiction and several health concerns. If you're struggling with tobacco use, you can also look for help from a professional.

Effects on Your Mood

Anxiety

Anxiety is a common effect of stress. This is when you feel nervous, tense, or afraid, and it can be accompanied by physical symptoms like a racing heart, sweating, and trembling. If you're feeling anxious, take a moment to relax and ease your anxiety. Meditation, breathing exercises, and yoga can all be helpful in reducing anxiety.

Irritability

Irritability is when you feel easily annoyed or angered, which can lead to arguments or fights with others. You may notice that you're more impatient than usual as well or quick to "snap." If you're feeling irritable, take a second to recalibrate and de-stress. Exercise, meditation, and deep breathing can reduce irritability.

Restlessness

Restlessness is when you feel you can't sit still or focus on anything. You may feel you're "jumpy" or "on edge." If you're feeling restless, it's important to relax and de-stress. Exercise, yoga, and walks in nature can reduce restlessness.

Angry Outbursts

Stress can lead to angry outbursts. This is when you feel you're suddenly furious and might lash out at others. For instance, you might yell at someone or throw your favorite lamp. If you're feeling like you might have an angry outburst, practice self-soothing techniques.

Lack of Motivation or Focus

Lack of motivation or focus is a common effect of anxiety. This is when you can't seem to focus on anything or get anything done. You may feel you're "spacing out" or "zoning out." If you're having trouble with motivation or focus, it's important to increase your motivation. Setting small goals, breaking up tasks into smaller chunks, and using a planner can all help you increase your motivation and focus.

Feeling Overwhelmed

Feeling overwhelmed is common when faced with stress. This is when you feel you can't handle anything or like everything is too much. You may feel you're "drowning" in your stress. If you're feeling overwhelmed, it's important to reduce your stress. Making a list of your tasks, setting priorities, and taking breaks can all help you feel less overwhelmed.

Chapter 3:

Is Your Lifestyle to Blame?

Are you angry all the time? Do you find yourself snapping at your loved ones, or getting into arguments with strangers for no reason? If so, your lifestyle might have a significant role in how you're feeling.

Think about it—are you getting enough sleep? Are you eating a balanced diet? Do you have regular downtime to relax and de-stress? Are you surrounded by negative people or struggling to find social support? If you answered "no" to any of the questions, it's no wonder you might feel on edge all the time. It might be time to re-evaluate your lifestyle and see if there are any changes you can make to help you feel calmer and more in control.

But don't worry, there's hope! Just by making a few minor changes to your lifestyle, you can see a big difference in how you're feeling. A holistic approach to managing your anger starts with examining your lifestyle. If you aren't taking care of yourself, it's going to be difficult to manage your emotions healthily.

How Do You Express Yourself Right Now?

Do you keep your anger bottled until it explodes? Or do you lash out and say things you later regret? Do you break things or hit people? What are your primary coping methods? Maybe you distance yourself from those who care for you and those you care for. Or maybe you turn to drugs or alcohol to help you numb the pain.

None of these methods are effective in managing your anger. There are healthier ways to express it; ways that won't damage your relationships or get you into legal trouble. It's important to find an outlet for your anger that works for you.

It's important to understand how you currently deal with your anger, as this will give you some insight into how to better manage it. If you're not sure where to start, begin by writing a list of all the things you do when you're feeling angry. If you're comfortable enough with your friends and family, ask them for their opinion too.

Sometimes, it's helpful to see your anger as a physical entity. What does it look like? Is it a big, hulking monster, or a small, sly fox? How does it make you feel? Is it hot or cold? Does it have a voice?

Spending some time to really understand your anger can help you better manage it. Once you know what sets it off and how it manifests, you can put some strategies in place to help you deal with it in a more constructive way.

How Did You Learn to Express Yourself?

Your anger didn't just appear out of nowhere—it's likely that you've been carrying it around for a long time. It might result from build-up from a lifetime of small slights and grievances, or it might be something that's only started to bother you recently. Think about how you learned to deal with your anger.

Were you taught to bottle it up? To never express your true feelings? Or, were you encouraged to lash out and express yourself in whatever way you saw fit? It's likely that your current coping mechanisms result from what you learned when growing up. If you were never taught how to deal with anger constructively, it can be tough to know where to start.

Or maybe your parents or caregivers struggled with their anger and that was the only example you had to employ. It's never too late to learn how to manage your anger. Even if you've been carrying around your anger for years, you can make a difference.

However, it's important to understand that you can learn new ways to express yourself. Just because you were taught to deal with your anger in a certain way, doesn't mean that's the only way you can do it.

What Is Your Social Circle Like Now?

Your social circle plays a big role in how you express your anger. If you're constantly surrounded by people who are angry and aggressive, it's difficult to find a different way to express yourself. If the people you associate with are negative and destructive, it's hard to break out of that mindset. On the other hand, if you're surrounded by people who are calm and supportive, it can have a positive influence on you and make it easier to find healthier ways to express your anger. Consider the people you spend the most time with and how they might affect your anger management.

Do You Have Any Support Systems in Place?

When you're feeling angry, it's helpful to have a support system in place—whether that's a friend, family member, therapist, or counselor. These people can provide a sounding board for you to express your anger in a safe and constructive way. They can also offer impartial advice and help you see things from a different perspective. If you don't have anyone you feel comfortable talking to about your anger, there are plenty of support groups and counseling services available that can help.

Chapter 4:

The Different Emotions at Play

What? You didn't think there was just one emotion in place of anger, did you? Oh no, there's a whole range of feelings that can come up and contribute to your anger. And they can all be just as intense, if not more so. Let's explore some of the different emotions that might be behind your anger.

Primary and Secondary Emotions

There are two types of emotions that can be at play when you're feeling angry: primary and secondary. Primary emotions are the ones that are directly related to the event or situation that's causing your anger. So, if someone veers in front of you in traffic, your primary emotion might be frustration. On the other hand, secondary emotions are feelings that arise in response to the primary emotion. So, with being cut off in traffic, your secondary emotions might be anxiety or fear.

The Different Types of Anger

There are different kinds of anger, each with its own set of contributing emotions.

Here are common types of anger:

- **Hostile**. This anger is characterized by feelings of hostility, meanness, and resentment. Emotions that might contribute to hostile anger include jealousy, envy, and hatred.

- **Displaced**. This type of anger is when you take your frustration out on someone who wasn't the original source of your anger. Emotions that can contribute to displaced anger include anxiety, stress, and fear.

- **Passive-aggressive anger**. This is when you express your anger in a passive-aggressive way, such as sarcasm or giving silent treatment. Emotions that might contribute to passive-aggressive anger include insecurity, resentment, and jealousy.

- **Volatile anger**. This is characterized by outbursts of anger that are often disproportionate to the event or situation. Emotions that can contribute to volatile anger include anxiety, stress, and fear.

- **Frustration-based**. This anger is motivated by feelings of frustration, such as when you're stuck in traffic or dealing with a difficult situation.

- **Pain-based**. This anger is in response to physical or emotional pain. Emotions that can contribute to pain-based anger include hurt, sadness, and fear.

- **Judgmental**. This anger is characterized by feelings of judgment, such as when you feel someone has wronged you. Emotions that can contribute to judgmental anger include resentment, bitterness, and grudges.

- **Manipulative anger**. This anger is expressed in a way that tries to control or manipulate the other person. Emotions that can contribute to manipulative anger include insecurity, neediness, and fear.

- **Physiological**. This anger results from a physical response, such as when you're hungry or tired. Emotions that can contribute to physiological anger include irritation, frustration, and anxiety.

- **Righteous**. This anger is characterized by feelings of being right or justified in your anger. Emotions that can contribute to righteous anger include indignation, self-righteousness, and moral superiority.

- **Retaliatory**. This anger is in response to someone else's aggression. Emotions that can contribute to retaliatory anger include fear, anxiety, and self-defense.

- **Overwhelmed anger**. This anger results from feeling overwhelmed, such as when you're dealing with a lot of stress. Emotions that can contribute to overwhelmed anger include anxiety, stress, and frustration.

- **Chronic anger**. This is long-term anger that's often the result of unresolved issues. Emotions that can contribute to chronic anger include resentment, bitterness, and grudges.

While this list isn't exhaustive, it does cover some of the most common types of anger, but not all of them will be present in every instance of anger. And, of course, there can be other emotions that contribute to anger that aren't listed here. It's also important to note that not all of these emotions are negative. For example, righteous anger can motivate you to take action against injustice. And chronic anger can be a sign that you need to make some changes in your life. What's important to remember is that there's no one right or wrong way to feel anger. Everybody experiences and expresses anger differently. And that's okay.

Anger and Its Other Emotions

Now that we've gone over the different anger, let's explore some of the other emotions that might be behind your anger:

- **Bitterness**. This is when you've been hurt by someone or something and you just can't let it go. You dwell on it and it festers inside of you until it comes out as anger. If you're feeling bitter, try to let go of the grudge. It's not worth holding onto and it's only going to hurt you in the end.

- **Resentment**. This is like bitterness, but it's usually directed towards someone who you feel has wronged you in some way. Maybe they did something that hurt you or they didn't do something that you think they should have done. Whatever the case may be, resentment is a poisonous emotion, and it's important to let it go.

- **Jealousy.** This emotion occurs when you feel like someone has something that you want and you get angry because of it. Maybe your friend just got a new car and you're jealous because you can't afford one right now. Or maybe your co-worker got a promotion and you're feeling stuck in your current position. Jealousy is a destructive emotion, and it's important to deal with it in a healthy way.

- **Envy.** This is like jealousy, but it's more focused on wanting what someone else has. Maybe you see your friend's happy marriage and you wish you had that in your own life. Or maybe you see someone's successful business and you wish you could be in their shoes. Envy is a dangerous emotion because it can lead to bitterness and resentment. It's important to be mindful of your envy and try to focus on the positive things in your own life.

- **Fear.** This is a common emotion that can cause anger. Maybe you're afraid of losing your job or your home. Or maybe you're afraid of being alone. Fear can be a powerful emotion, and dealing with it healthily is crucial for managing anger.

- **Anxiety**. This is another common emotion that can cause anger. Maybe you're anxious about an upcoming test or presentation. Or maybe you're anxious about your future. Anxiety can be a very debilitating emotion.

- **Disbelief**. This is when you can't believe what's happening or you don't believe that someone is telling the truth. It's like you're in a dream and you just want to wake up. Maybe you're in disbelief that your boss just fired you. Or maybe you're in disbelief that your partner just cheated on you. Disbelief can be a very confusing emotion and it needs to be released properly.

- **Sadness**. This is another emotion that can cause anger. Maybe you're feeling sad because you lost your job or your home. Or maybe you're feeling sad because a loved one died. Sadness is a very difficult emotion to deal with, but coping with it will make it easier to overcome.

There are many emotions that can cause anger, but these are some of the most common ones. It's important to be aware of the emotions that you're feeling and to deal with them healthily. If you're not sure how to do that, there are many additional resources available to help you. Anger is a normal emotion, but it can be destructive if it's not managed properly.

Displaced Anger

Sometimes, people might feel angry but they don't know why. This is called displaced anger. Displaced anger is when you take your anger out on someone or something that isn't the source of your anger. This often occurs when you're angry at someone or something, but you can't or don't want to express it directly.

Maybe you're angry with your boss, but you can't say anything because you need your job. So, you go home and take it out on your spouse. Or maybe you're angry at your partner, but you don't want to start a fight. Displaced anger can be destructive because it can lead to passive-aggressive behavior, which can be harmful to your relationships. It's important to deal with your anger healthily so that you don't take it out on the wrong person.

Chapter 5:

Understanding Your Triggers

We all have triggers. You know, those things that just set us off for no reason? Maybe it's a certain type of person or a certain situation. Maybe it's something someone says or does. Whatever it is, we all have our triggers, and they can be tough to deal with. But the thing is, if we can understand our triggers, we can learn to control our reactions to them. We can learn to calm our anger and avoid getting into situations that we'll regret later.

What Are Triggers?

A trigger is anything that sets off a memory or reaction in the body. It can be a person, place, thing, or situation. It can also be a smell, taste, sound, or sight. Triggers are often associated with traumatic events. For example, a person who has been in a car accident might have a fear of driving.

Or, a person who was sexually abused might have a fear of being touched. Triggers can also be associated with difficult life transitions, such as moving to a new city or starting a new job. Some triggers are positive and can help us feel happy, loved, and supported. Other triggers are negative and can cause us to feel anxious, angry, or scared.

Types of Triggers

There are two types of triggers: internal and external.

Internal triggers are thoughts, or memories that are stored in the mind. They can be positive or negative. For example, a memory of a loved one who has passed away might make us feel sad. Or, a memory of a happy childhood experience might make us feel happy.

External triggers are anything in the environment that can trigger a memory or reaction. They can be people, places, things, or situations. For example, seeing a dog that used to look like one we had that passed away can make us feel sad. Or, going to a place where we had an exciting experience might make us feel happy.

Who Are You?

An important part of determining your triggers is figuring out who you are. This includes understanding your values, beliefs, and identity. When you know who you are, it's easier to figure out what sets you off. Are you the type of person who gets angry easily? Why? What sets you off? Your triggers can be a person, place, thing, situation, or anything that elicits a negative response from you.

They can be people, places, things, situations, or even thoughts. Perhaps you have a trigger that sets off a memory of a traumatic event. Or maybe you get angry when someone challenges your beliefs. Once you know what sets you off, it's easier to figure out why.

The next step is to figure out why your triggers have the power to set you off. Is it the way someone looks at you? Is it the tone of their voice? Or is it something they say? Once you've identified your triggers, you'll be one step closer to learning how to control your reactions to them. Once you know what your triggers are, it's time to work on controlling your reactions to them.

How to Handle Triggers

The best way to handle a trigger is to identify it and then cope with it. Coping with a trigger can be difficult, but it's important to remember that you have the power to control your reaction to it. There are a few methods that you can use to cope with triggers:

- **Identify your triggers**. The first step is to identify your triggers. This can be difficult, but being aware of what sets off your reactions can help you pinpoint your major pain points.

- **Avoid your triggers**. If possible, avoid your triggers. This isn't always possible, but it's helpful to avoid situations you know will be difficult for you. For example, if you have a fear of driving, you might avoid getting in the car. Or, if you have a fear of being around people, you might avoid social situations. While avoidance can lead to more significant problems down the road, in the short term, it can help you cope with your triggers.

- **Use positive coping strategies**. Aside from the distraction methods mentioned above, some people use positive coping strategies, such as deep or focused breathing techniques, progressive muscle relaxation, or meditation. Others use distraction techniques, such as listening to music or watching a movie. Some might use journaling or art to express their feelings. Experiment with a variety of mechanisms to see what works best for you.

- **Prepare for your triggers**. If you can't avoid your triggers, it's important to be prepared for them. This means knowing what you'll do when you face a trigger. For example, if you have a fear of driving, you might plan to take a different route that doesn't involve getting on the highway. Or, if you're nervous about being around people, you might plan to bring a friend with you to social situations.

- **Talk to someone**. Triggers can be difficult to deal with on your own. If you're struggling to cope with your triggers, it's important to talk to someone who can help. This might be a therapist, counselor, or other mental health professional.

What Not to Do

A few common challenges can arise when you're faced with a trigger that you should avoid. First, don't push through your fear or anxiety. For instance, if you're afraid of public speaking, don't force yourself to do it without preparing yourself. This will only make it worse. Second, don't suppress your emotions, such as keeping your anger locked up tightly within. This can be tough, but allow yourself to feel your emotions freely. Lastly, don't rationalize your way out of your feelings. For example, don't tell yourself that you shouldn't be feeling anxious because there's nothing to be anxious about. This will only make you feel worse.

What Are Some Common Triggers?

There are several things that can trigger a memory or reaction. Here are some of the most common triggers:

- **People**. People can be a major trigger for many people. This might be a specific person, such as a parent or ex-partner. Or, it might be a group of people, such as women or men.

- **Places**. Places can also be a major trigger for many people. This might be a specific place, such as a home or workplace. Or, it might be a type of place, such as a school or hospital.

- **Things.** Things or objects can be a trigger for many people. This might be a specific thing, such as a car or toy. Or, it might be a picture or sound.

- **Senses.** A trigger might be a specific sense, such as sight or sound. Or, it might be a combination of senses, such as smell and taste.

- **Emotions.** A trigger for many people can also be specific emotions. This might be a specific emotion, such as anger or sadness. Or, it might be a type of emotion, such as fear or anxiety.

Avoid Provocations

When you're trying to calm your anger, it's important to avoid provocation. This means avoiding things that might make you angry. Here are some tips:

- **Self-counseling**. If you're feeling angry, look at the situation as a whole and assess it appropriately. This means looking at the facts and trying to see things from different perspectives.

- **Empathize with the person who angered you**. It's helpful to change your perspective to understand the situation from the other person's point of view. Agreeing with them isn't necessary, but it can help you understand why they might have acted the way they did.

Find Solutions to Social Problems

When trying to calm your anger, it's important to also try and find solutions to social problems. This means working towards objectives that can help make the world a stronger environment.

Styles of Social Problem-Solving

People handle problems in different ways. Here are a few common problem-solving styles:

- **An impulsive, careless style**. You act without thinking about the consequences of your actions.
- **An avoidant style**. You try to avoid social problems altogether.
- **A positive style**. You try to find a solution that works for everyone involved.

Positive Problem-Solving

This style of problem-solving is based on the belief that there's a solution that can be found that will work for everyone involved. When using this style, it's important to:

- **Define the problem**. The first step is to identify the problem.
- **Generate potential solutions**. Once the problem is identified, it's time to brainstorm workable solutions. This means thinking about what might work to solve the problem.
- **Choose the best solution**. After generating potential solutions, it's time to choose the best one. This means looking at the pros and cons of each solution and selecting the plan that will work best for everyone involved.

Negative Problem-Solving

This problem-solving technique is based on the thought that there's no well-rounded solution. Negative problem-solving skills can cause:

- **Destructive conflict**. When using this style, it's more likely that conflict will become destructive. This means that people will fight and argue with each other, instead of creating a solution together.
- **Gridlock**. This is when a problem gets stuck and no progress is made. This can happen when people are only focused on their own needs and are not willing to compromise.

Steps of Social Problem-Solving

The steps of social problem-solving are:

1. **Clearly state the concern**. The first step is to identify the concerns within the situation.

2. **Invite others to share their thoughts**. Once the problem is identified, it's important to involve others in finding a solution. This means asking for input from others and considering their ideas.

3. **Generate several workable solutions**. Once the problem is identified and others have been involved, it's time to brainstorm potential solutions. This means thinking about what might solve the problem.

4. **Determine what are the immediate side effects**. It's important to consider the potential consequences of each solution before deciding on the best one.

5. **Determine the long-term side effects**. Besides looking at the immediate consequences of a solution, it's also important to consider the long-term effects. This means thinking about how a solution will impact people in the future.

6. **Create and implement the best course of action**. Once the best solution has been chosen, it's time to put it into action. This means creating a plan and then taking steps to implement it.

7. **Monitor the situation**. After a solution has been put into action, it's important to monitor the situation to make sure it's working. This means paying attention to how the problem is changing and adjusting the solution as needed.

8. **Analyze your response**. It's also important to reflect on your own behavior during the problem-solving process. This means thinking about what you did well and what you could improve on for next time.

So, what are your triggers? Make a list of them. Once you've got them down on paper, look at each one, and try to figure out what it is about that trigger that sets you off. Is it the looks people give you? Is it the tone of their voice? Or is it something they say?

Now that you're aware of your triggers, it's time to start working on controlling your reactions to them. This can be tough, but it's important to remember that you always have a choice in how you react to a situation. You can choose to let your anger take over, or you can choose to stay calm. It might not be easy, but with practice, you can learn to control your reactions and keep your anger in check.

When you're feeling calm, it's much easier to think clearly and make morally sound decisions. So the next time you're feeling angry, take a deep breath and try to remember that you always choose how you react. Choose to stay calm, and you'll be one step closer to mastering your anger.

Chapter 6:

Understanding Your End Goal

When you're angry, try to determine what your end goal is. Are you trying to hurt the person who wronged you? Are you trying to get them to admit they were wrong? Are you trying to make them feel as angry as you do? Your end goal will dictate how you go about expressing your anger. If your goal is to hurt the other person, then you'll likely lash out aggressively.

If your goal is to get them to admit to your viewpoint, you'll likely try to reason with them. If your goal is to make them feel angry as well, then you'll likely try to provoke them. Not all goals are equal. Some goals, like trying to hurt the other person, are more likely to lead to negative outcomes than others. If your goal is to inflict pain on the other person, it's important to consider whether that's really something you want to do. You may find that there are better ways to obtain your goals.

Why Are You Angry?

Before you can cope with your anger, it's important to understand why you're feeling angry in the first place.

There are a few different reasons people get angry:

- **Someone has hurt you**. If someone has physically or emotionally hurt you, it's natural to feel angry. You may feel you need to lash out in order to protect yourself.

- **Someone has wronged you**. If someone has done something that you perceive as being wrong, it's natural to feel angry. You may feel you need to set things right.

- **You're stressed**. If you're under a lot of stress, it's natural to feel angry. You may feel you can't cope with everything that's going on in your life.

- **You're tired**. If you're tired, it's natural to feel angry. You may feel you can't do anything right. People are angered for a variety of reasons.

Pinpoint the Goal of Your Anger

As we mentioned before, it's important to understand the goal of your anger. Are you trying to hurt the other person? Do you want them to admit to their wrongdoings? Do you want them to be as angry as you are? Does the situation remind you of a previous hurt? Once you've identified the goal of your anger, you'll be in a better position to deal with it.

What Is Your Anger Trying to Tell You?

It's important to understand that anger is a normal emotion. It's not necessarily a bad thing. In fact, anger can be a positive force in your life. It can motivate you to take action and make changes. It can also help you grasp your wants and needs. If you're feeling angry, it's important to take a step back and ask yourself what your anger is trying to tell you. What do you need to do in order to feel better? Do you need to confront the person who hurt you? Do you need to take some time for yourself? Once you've identified what your anger is trying to convey, you'll have a better idea of how to deal with it.

Then you have to consider how the other person is feeling. They might be angry because they think you're trying to hurt them. If they're feeling defensive, it's likely because they think you're trying to get them to admit to their faults. If they're feeling scared, it's likely because they think you're trying to make them feel angry too. Be careful with your words and actions, so you don't make the situation worse. It's important to remain calm and collected, even if the other person isn't. The best way to deal with your anger is to understand why you're feeling it in the first place.

The Root of Anger

There are a few different theories about the root of anger. Some people understand anger is natural and that everyone experiences it. Others believe that anger is a learned response to certain situations. Yet, others believe that anger results from unresolved issues from the past. Various triggers can cause anger. The root of your anger will be unique to you. It's important to explore your own personal history and experiences in order to better understand the root of your anger.

Therapies and Understanding Your Anger

If you're having trouble managing your anger, there are a few different therapies that can help. Cognitive behavioral therapy (CBT) can help you understand the thoughts and behaviors that contribute to your anger. Dialectical behavioral therapy (DBT) can help you develop skills for dealing with difficult emotions. Eye movement desensitization and reprocessing (EMDR) can help you process and heal from past traumas.

Family therapy can also be very beneficial. If you have a close relationship with your family, they may help you understand and manage your anger. Find a therapist or counselor who you feel understands you and makes you comfortable. You should feel you can trust them and that they understand your needs.

Psychodynamic therapy may also be helpful. This type of therapy can help you understand the unconscious thoughts and feelings that contribute to your anger.

Therapy can help you understand your anger and develop skills for managing it.

In therapy you'll:

- examine the circumstances in your life that cultivate anger or stress
- understand how anger and stress negatively impact the quality of your life
- identify the triggers, thoughts, and emotions that contribute to your anger
- recognize and identify negative thought patterns or self-talk
- learn new responses to feelings of stress and anger that don't include aggression
- define and become aware of the range of stress and anger, and track your current levels
- develop a plan to deal with stressors as they arise in your daily life
- practice relaxation techniques to help you stay calm in the face of stress
- commit to making changes in your life that will support your anger management goals

Therapy can help you significantly; however, it's important to remember that change takes time. You won't be able to resolve all of your issues overnight. It's important to be patient and to commit to the process. If you're interested in exploring therapy, there are a few different ways to find a therapist.

You can ask your doctor for a referral, search online directories, or ask friends or family for recommendations. You don't have to wait until you're in the middle of a crisis to seek help. If you're struggling to manage your anger, reach out for help. It's never too early to start working on making changes in your life.

Chapter 7:

Balancing Your Life

To make the symptoms of anger easier to manage, you can focus on balancing your life and creating a well-rounded routine. This chapter reviews different tactics you can apply to balance your life to manage your anger.

Causes of an Unbalanced Life

There are many things that can cause an unbalanced life. Some of the most common include:

- **Age**. As we get older, our responsibilities tend to increase. If we're not careful about how we manage our life, we can become stressed.

- **Family**. This can be a source of both joy and stress. Find a balance between taking care of who we love and taking care of ourselves.

- **Work.** This can be a source of both satisfaction and frustration. Find a balance between your job and the rest of your life.

- **Money**. This can be a source of both security and anxiety. Have a balance between your financial needs and your desire to live a comfortable life.

- **Personality**. Everyone has their own unique personality. Some people are more prone to an unbalanced life than others. Maybe you're a people pleaser or a perfectionist. Maybe you have a fear of failure. Whatever the case may be, it's important to be aware of your personality and how it affects your life.

- **Overemphasis on independence**. In our society, there's a lot of emphasis on independence. We're taught to be self-sufficient and to take care of ourselves. While independence is important, it's also important to know when to ask for help. Otherwise, we'll take on too much.

- **Unrealistic expectations**. We live in a world that is full of unrealistic expectations. We're bombarded with images of flawless bodies, relationships, and lives. It's important to remember that these images are not real. They're airbrushed and Photoshopped. They're not achievable. When we compare our lives to these unrealistic standards, we can become overwhelmed.

- **Relying on unhealthy pleasures**. We all have activities we enjoy and engage in. These things can include food, TV, alcohol, drugs, sex, shopping, and gambling. While there's nothing wrong with enjoying these things in moderation, it can become a problem when we rely on them to make us happy. When we do this, we're choosing an unhealthy pleasure over a healthy one. We're choosing to numb our pain instead of dealing with it, which can lead to hidden triggers.

- **Not taking care of yourself**. It's important to take care of yourself, both physically and emotionally. When you don't, it can lead to an unbalanced life. Not taking care of yourself can lead to physical and emotional problems. It can make it harder to cope with stress. It can also lead to behaviors such as drinking excessive alcohol, smoking cigarettes, and engaging in drugs. Not taking care of yourself can include:
  - not eating healthy foods
  - not getting enough sleep
  - not exercising
  - not taking time for yourself
  - not having a support system

- **Stress**. Stress is a normal part of life. It's our body's way of responding to changes. While some stress can be helpful, too much stress can be harmful. When we're stressed, our body goes into fight-or-flight mode. This means that our body accommodates us by raising our heart rate, increasing blood pressure, and breathing more quickly. This response helps us deal with a threat. However, when we're constantly stressed, our body never returns to its normal state.

- **Technology**. Technology can be a great thing. It can connect us to other people, such as our loved ones, stay organized, and get information. However, it can also be a source of stress. When we're constantly connected to our devices, it's hard to disconnect from the outside world, which can leave us feeling unfulfilled.

- **Lack of perspective**. When we're bogged down by the day-to-day tasks of life, it's hard to see the big picture. We can get so caught up in our own lives that we forget about what's really important, which can cause us to prioritize the wrong things.

- **Lack of exercise**. Exercise is important for our physical and emotional health. When we don't exercise often, it can lead to other health problems.

- **Income to expenses ratio**. It's important to have a healthy relationship with money. When our income doesn't match our expenses, we can become stressed with financial woes.

- **Not having a support system**. We all need someone to lean on from time to time. When we don't have a support system, we don't know who to turn to, which can leave us feeling lonely and angry.

- **Not having goals**. It's important to have goals in life. Without goals, it's hard to know what we're working towards, which can cause us to fall behind.

- **No vacations**. Everyone needs the occasional break. When we don't take vacations, it can lead to an unbalanced life because we're constantly working and we're not giving ourselves a chance to relax.

Signs That You May Have an Unbalanced Life

There are many signs that you may have an unbalanced life. Some of these signs may be physical, while others may be emotional. If you're experiencing any of the following, it's a good idea to seek help:

- You're always tired.
- You're not taking care of yourself.
- You're always stressed.
- You're not enjoying life.
- You're not happy.
- You're not fulfilled.

Having balance in your life is important for managing anger. This means that you should have time for work, play, and rest. You should also have time for your relationships, interests, and mental and physical well-being. When we're out of balance, we're more likely to get stressed and angry. When you have balance in your life, you're less likely to feel overwhelmed and angry.

To maintain a healthy balance, it's important to:

- **Schedule regular check-ins with yourself.** This means taking some time each day, week, or month to check in with yourself. Ask yourself how you're feeling and what you need.

- **Make time for the things that are important to you**. This means putting aside time for people or activities that are important to you, like your relationships, hobbies, and well-being.

- **Say no to things that don't serve you**. This means learning to say no to things that don't fit into your life. This might include saying no to extra work, social obligations, or anything else that doesn't make you feel positive about the experience.

- **Create boundaries**. This means setting limits with others and learning to say no. It also means caring for yourself by implementing structured rest and relaxation.

Controlling Anger Equals Finding the Balance Between SNS and PNS

In order to control anger, find a balance between the SNS and PNS. When we're angry, our SNS is activated. However, the PNS can help us calm down. We can activate the PNS by doing things like concentrated, deep breathing, paired or progressive muscle relaxation, and guided or visual meditations. If you can trigger the PNS to overcome the SNS, you can help to control your anger.

You can stimulate the PNS by:

- **Practicing progressive muscle relaxation**. This involves tightening and relaxing different muscles throughout your body. Start by tensing the muscles in your toes for five seconds and then relax them. Work your way up to your neck and face muscles.

- **Deep breathing**. Take deep breaths from your stomach, not your chest. Breathe in through your nose and out through your mouth.

- **Meditation**. Try to focus on your breath and clear your mind of other thoughts.

- **Visualization**. Imagine a peaceful scene, such as a beach or a meadow.

- **Get moving**. Exercise can help to dissipate anger.

These techniques can help to calm your anger and give you a better sense of control. Try out different techniques to determine what helps you the most.

Counterbalancing Stress to Improve Our Health

We all experience stress, but too much stress can harm our health. When we're stressed, our bodies release cortisol, which can lead to physical and mental health problems. To counterbalance the effects of stress, it's important to:

- **Include positives in your life**. Share your time with people who make you feel positive and joyous. People who do things that make you happy, and focus on the benefits of life that are going well. Make time for relaxation: Take some time each day to relax and rejuvenate. This might include taking a warm bath, reading a book, or spending time in nature.

- **Reduce extremes**. Avoid situations that are too stressful or too stimulating. This might include watching the news, working long hours, or being around negative people.

- **Create healthy pleasure**. Experience joy and pleasure in your life. This might include listening to serene music, spending time with loved ones, or doing something that brings you peace. When we have healthy pleasure in our lives, it's easier to cope with stress and anger.

- **Maintain meaningful social ties**. Having strong social ties can improve your health. Social support can help reduce stress, strengthen mental and physical health, and even lengthen your life. Interacting with others and maintaining social ties can help you balance your life and manage your anger.

Start With Yourself First

The most important relationship you have is the one you have with yourself. When you're angry, it's easy to be hard on yourself. But being kind and understanding with yourself is an important part of managing anger. Try to:

- be patient with yourself

- accept your mistakes—everyone makes them
- practice self-compassion
- learn from your mistakes

Make Time for the Things You Love

When we're angry, it's easy to forget about the things we love. But setting aside time for activities you love is an important part of managing anger. Doing things you enjoy can help you relax, de-stress, and make you feel connected to something outside of yourself. Make sure to:

- schedule time for the things you love
- stick to your schedule
- be flexible—if something comes up, don't be afraid to change your plans

Check Your Thoughts

When we're angry, our thoughts can be negative and distorted. This can affect those we spend our time with as well. Checking your thoughts means being aware of the things you're thinking and how they're affecting your mood. If you notice your thoughts are negative, review the facts to make sure your beliefs are accurate. If your thoughts are inaccurate, they can make your anger worse. Try to:

- question your thoughts
- look at the evidence
- challenge your beliefs
- practice positive thinking

Get Outside and Step Out of Your Mind

Sometimes, the best way to calm your anger is to get outside and away from the situation. This can help you clear your head and see the challenge from a new perspective. It can also prompt you to get some much-needed physical activity. Don't allow yourself to stay stuck in your anger. You might meet unique people and create deep, meaningful connections with others. Get up and move around. Go for a walk, take a yoga class, or just go outside to breathe in the crisp air.

Choose Your Battles

It's important to pick your battles when you're angry. Not every situation is worth getting upset about. If the situation isn't important, let it go. Choose your battles wisely. Otherwise, you'll end up expending energy and wasting time on things that don't matter.

Be Proactive

When developing meaningful relationships, it's important to be proactive. This means reaching out to others and fostering connections. It can also mean being assertive in your interactions. Being proactive can help you build sturdy, long-term relationships and prevent conflict. Additionally, if you feel your anger rising when you're with others, don't wait for it to boil over before you deal with it. Be proactive about managing your anger. This means taking steps to prevent it before it starts. It also means dealing with anger as soon as it arises. The sooner you deal with it, the easier it is to manage.

Be Present

When you're with others, be present. This means being fully engaged in the moment. It means being aware of your thoughts, feelings, and actions. It also means being aware of the thoughts, feelings, and actions of those around you. Being present can help you build a bond with others and avoid miscommunications. Additionally, it can help you be more understanding and compassionate when dealing with others.

Make Time For Yourself

A great way to combat an unbalanced life is to make time for yourself. Caring for yourself can build up your self-esteem, which makes it easier to deal with stress. Your confidence becomes enhanced, making it easier to take on new challenges. Plus, practicing self-care releases endorphins, which have mood-boosting properties.

Self-care doesn't have to be time-consuming or expensive. There are many simple things you can do to take care of yourself. Here are some ideas:

- **Get enough sleep**. Sleep is crucial for our well-being. Make sure you're getting enough sleep every night.
- **Exercise**. Exercise releases endorphins, which have mood-boosting properties.

- **Eat healthy**. Eating healthy foods helps our bodies function properly.
- **Take breaks**. When you're feeling overwhelmed, take a few minutes to yourself to relax.
- **Do something you enjoy**. Pencil activities you enjoy into your schedule. This will help you relax and de-stress.
- **Create a morning routine**. Start your day off right with a morning routine that sets a positive tone for the rest of the day. Consider all the activities you do in the morning and create a schedule that works for you and helps you prepare for the rest of the day. This might include meditation, journaling, or exercise.
- **Create an evening routine**. Just like a morning routine, an evening routine will help you wind down at the end of the day and prepare for sleep. This might include reading, taking a bath, or writing in a journal. You can also use this time to gather what you'll need for the following day, so you're not rushed in the morning.
- **Make time for your hobbies**. Hobbies are a great way to relax and de-stress. Make sure you're making time for your hobbies like painting, hiking, biking, or whatever it is you enjoy.

Chapter 8:

Ways of Coping With and Controlling Anger

Sometimes, anger takes a hold of us more easily than we'd like. If you struggle to keep it in check, you have a variety of options to regain control. Some people may need to intertwine multiple methods to find what works best for them. However, by having a few tools in your arsenal, you're more likely to be successful in keeping your anger under control.

Distress Tolerance—DBT Skills

This skill set helps you tolerate and manage overwhelming emotions and situations. The skills in this set can be very helpful when you're struggling with intense emotions, like anger.

Distress tolerance can be a tough challenge to overcome. Luckily, there are several acronyms in place to help you remember what to do. One acronym to remember is **ACCEPTS**, which stands for activities, contributing, comparisons, emotions, pushing away, thoughts, and sensations (Linehan, n.d.-b):

- **A—Activities**. Engage in an activity to take your mind off of the situation that's causing your anger.
- **C—Contributing**. Help others by volunteering or doing something nice for someone else.
- **C—Comparisons**. Comparing the current situation to other situations in order to put it into perspective. When have you felt worse and how did you overcome it? How could the situation be more challenging?
- **E—Recognize and label your emotions**. This can help you understand and manage them better.
- **P—Pushing away.** Instead of dwelling in a never-ending loop of negative thoughts, look for something positive to focus on and push away those self-stigmas.
- **T—Thoughts.** Be mindful of your thoughts and try to reframe them in a more positive light.
- **S—Sensations.** Pay attention to your body and how it's reacting to the situation. This can help you catch yourself before you get too angry.

Another acronym to help you is **TIPP**, which stands for temperature, intense exercise, paced breathing, and paired muscle relaxation (Greene, 2020):

- **T–Temperature**. Change the temperature of your environment or take a cold shower to help cool down your body and mind. Altering your body's temperature can help change your mood.
- **I—Intense exercise**. Getting your heart rate up through intense exercise can help you burn off that excess energy and anger.
- **P—Paced breathing**. Try to take slow and deep breaths in through your nose. Blow out

through your mouth. This can help center you and calm you down.

- **P—Paired muscle relaxation**. Start by tensing up your muscles as much as you can and then releasing them. Work your way through your whole body until you feel more relaxed.

Another acronym is IMPROVE, which stands for imagery, meaning, prayer, relaxation, one thing in the moment, vacation, and encouragement (Linehan, n.d.-g):

- **I—Imagery**. Use your imagination to picture a calming scene or happy memory. This can help you redirect your mind from the situation that's causing your anger.

- **M—Meaning**. Try to find meaning in the situation. What can you learn from this? How can you grow from this?

- **P—Prayer**. If you're religious or spiritual, prayer can be a helpful way to calm your anger. If you're not religious, taking a few moments to speak out loud, meditating, or closing your eyes and rid your mind of what's bothering you can help you calm down.

- **R—Relaxation**. As we mentioned before, relaxation techniques can be helpful in managing your anger. Try deep breathing, aromatherapy, or progressive muscle relaxation.

- **O—One thing in the moment**. Focus on one thing that you can control in the situation. This could be your own actions or how you're feeling. Find relief in that one thing.

- **V—Vacation**. Take a mental or a physical break from the situation. Go for a walk, workout, listen to your favorite music, or read a book. Visit a new country, travel to another state, or rent a cabin in the woods. Do something that you enjoy to take your mind off of your triggers.

- **E—Encouragement**. Offer yourself encouragement by speaking kindly to yourself. This can help you feel relaxed and in control of your abilities.

These are just a few of the many acronyms and skills that can help you calm your anger. While these skills can be helpful, they may need to be tweaked to work well for you. What works for you may not work for others. Find the techniques that work best for you and practice regularly.

Practicing Radical Acceptance

One of the most important things that you can do to calm your anger is to practice radical acceptance. This means accepting things as they are, even if they're not what you want them to be. Radical acceptance doesn't mean that you're happy with the situation, but it does mean that you're accepting it as it is.

This can be a difficult skill to practice, but it's important to remember that acceptance doesn't mean that you're giving up. It's okay to still want things to be different, but acceptance can help you move on from the anger and negativity that you're feeling.

Try to remember that not everything in life is going to go how you want it to. This is normal, and it's okay. Don't get too caught up in the things that you can't control. Instead, concentrate on what is in your control, like your responses and emotions.

Some tips to remember when practicing radical acceptance:

- Radical acceptance means complete or total—it doesn't mean half-hearted.
- Rejecting reality doesn't change it.
- There are limits to the future.
- Everything has a cause.
- Pain can't be avoided, but life is worth living.

If you can remember these things, it will be easier for you to accept the things that you can't control. And when you're able to accept the things that you can't control, you'll find that your anger will start to dissipate.

In the Moment Cool Down Techniques

Leave the Situation

You can just leave the situation to calm yourself, deal with your emotions, and then return to deal with things more rationally. When you experience physiological signs of rage, you might need to take action like this. This is probably the most effective thing you can do, but it's not always possible.

For instance, you might be in the middle of a meeting at work, or you might be in the middle of an argument with your spouse. But if you can, just walking away can be the best solution. This gives you time to calm down and to think about how you really want to handle the situation.

Change Your Thoughts

Our thoughts influence our emotions and behaviors. So if you're thinking angry thoughts, it's likely that you'll feel angry. However, by changing your thought process, you can improve your emotional state.

For instance, if you're thinking, "That person is so stupid! I can't believe they did that!" you're likely to feel angry. But if you change your thought to, "That person isn't thinking clearly. I wonder what's going on with them," you're likely to feel compassion instead of anger.

Relaxation Techniques and Meditation

Both relaxation techniques and meditation can relax your mind, soul, and body. When you're relaxed, your body is in a different physiological state than when you're angry, which is incompatible. Exercises can help the state of relaxation to be dominant, so you can handle the situation appropriately.

Progressive muscle relaxation is just one example of a relaxation technique. In this technique, you tense particular muscle groups for a set time. Then relax and release the pain with it. You repeat this throughout your body, which reduces the stress and tension stored in your body. Mindfulness meditation is another relaxation technique. In mindfulness meditation, your awareness is in your breath and the present moment. This helps you notice how your thoughts and emotions affect you but release them without the infliction of self-judgment.

Convince Yourself to Calm Down

Sometimes talking to yourself in a calm, soothing voice can help release tension. This is especially true if you're feeling physiological signs of rage, like a racing heart or clenched fists. You might say something like, "It's okay. Calm down. Everything is going to be alright." Or you might say, "Take a deep breath. Inhale and count to four. Exhale and count down from four."

Convince yourself to do it. Talk to yourself and use logic to convince yourself to become more composed. Positive self-talk techniques include reminding oneself not to take things personally, that the current situation isn't indicative of the rest of one's life, and focusing on problem-solving instead of dwelling on the problem itself.

Use Humor

Humor can be a great way to diffuse anger. If you can laugh at the situation, you're likely to feel less angry. Of course, this isn't always appropriate. If someone has done something that has really hurt you, laughing it off probably won't be helpful. But if you're in a minor disagreement with someone, or if you're feeling angry about a situation that isn't really that serious, humor can be a great way to calm down.

You can focus on the ridiculousness of the situation, or you can try to come up with a funny solution to the problem. This technique won't work for everyone, but if you're the type of person who responds well to humor, it can help you loosen up.

Resolving Conflict

Express Your Emotions Effectively

If you're feeling angry, it's important to express your emotions in a way that is assertive, but not aggressive. This means that you should speak up for yourself, but you shouldn't try to put the other person down. Assertive communication is based on respect, both for yourself and for the other person. You have a right to your feelings and opinions, but so does the other person.

If you're feeling angry, try to use "I" statements. For instance, you might say, "I'm feeling furious right now." This will convey to the other person how you're feeling without being aggressive or attacking them.

Practice Active Listening Skills

Active listening is a way of communication that involves fully understanding what the other person is saying. Listen carefully to what the other person is saying. This is more important than trying to win an argument.

Try to rephrase the other person's point to make sure that you understand. For instance, you might say, "So, you're feeling really frustrated because you feel like I'm not listening to you." Do not interrupt. Allow the other person to fully express themselves before you respond.

Try to empathize with the other person. Empathy is the ability to understand how the other person is feeling. You don't have to agree with their viewpoint, but make an effort to understand their concerns. Consider why they feel the way they do. For instance, you might say, "I can see how you would feel that way." Or, "It makes sense that you would be angry in this situation." This will help the other person to feel heard and understood.

Negotiate or Compromise When Necessary

In some situations, it might not be possible to come to a resolution that satisfies everyone. In these cases, it's important to negotiate or compromise.

Negotiation is a process of give and take, where both parties try to come to an agreement that is acceptable to both. Compromise is like negotiation, but it usually involves each person giving up something in order to come to an agreement. Both techniques can be helpful in situations where it's not possible to find a resolution that everyone is happy with and is a vital part of healthy communication.

Use DEAR MAN

DEAR MAN is an acronym used in DBT to help people effectively communicate their needs. It stands for:

- **D**escribe the situation.

- **E**xpress your emotions about the situation and why it's a concern for you.
- **A**ssert your needs or wants—make it clear what you're asking for.
- **R**einforce or reward the other person—explain to them the benefits they would receive.
- **M**indful of the situation, yourself, and the other person—focus on the goal and don't let distractions get the best of you.
- **A**ppear confident—use a calm and confident tone of voice.
- **N**egotiate—be willing to give and take in order to come to an agreement (*Common dialectical behavior therapy DBT acronyms*, 2018).

Other Helpful Techniques

There are several other techniques that can be helpful when dealing with anger. Try to find methods that are beneficial for you and use them when you're feeling angry.

Some other helpful techniques include the following.

Recognize the Warning Signs

Take some time to learn your body's warning signs you're getting angry. This will help you take steps to calm down before you get too angry. Some common warning signs of anger include feeling tense, feeling hot, having a fast heart rate, clenching your fists or teeth, and feeling like you're going to explode. If you notice any of these warning signs, take a few deep breaths and try to calm down.

Understand Your Anger

Work out why you're angry. This can be helpful in learning how to deal with your anger healthily. This will help you deal with the root of the problem, rather than just the symptoms.

There are several things that can cause anger. Some common causes include feeling like you're not being heard or respected, feeling like you're being treated unfairly, feeling frustrated, feeling helpless or powerless, and feeling threatened.

Write It Out

Writing can be a beneficial way to deal with anger. It can help you express your thoughts and feelings constructively. Writing can also help you make sense of your anger and figure out what's causing it.

Try writing about what happened, how you're feeling, and why you're angry. You might also want to write about what you'd like to happen or how you'd like the situation to be resolved. When you're finished, walk away for a little and then reread it when you've calmed down. This break will give you time to view the situation clearly and make better decisions about how to deal with your anger.

Count to 100

Sometimes, all you need is a little time to calm down. If you're feeling angry, try counting to 100 slowly. This will help to distract you and give you time to calm down. Once you've reached 100, reassess the situation or check in with yourself to see how you feel.

Press Pause

In the heat of the moment, it's often hard to make healthy decisions. If you're feeling angry, try taking a step back from the situation. Mentally picture yourself pressing the "pause" button on a remote control in your hand. You can use this time to calm down and think more clearly about how to deal with the situation. Once you're relaxed, you can return and deal with the situation in a more constructive way.

Move Around

Physical activity can help to release some of the tension you're feeling. If you're feeling angry, try going for a walk, run, or swim. You might also want to try some deep breathing exercises or stretching.

Talk to Someone

Talking to someone can help you deal with anger. They can help you see the situation from a different perspective and offer helpful suggestions. It can also be helpful to just talk about what's going on and how you're feeling. You can express your thoughts and feelings constructively. Sometimes, just saying it out loud can help to make it feel less overwhelming.

Take Time for Yourself

If you're feeling angry, sometimes, it's helpful to take some time for yourself. This can be a time to calm down, relax, and think about what's going on.

Biofeedback

Many people think that the only way to deal with anger is to let it all out, but that's not true. In fact, sometimes it's better to keep your cool and use some self-control. One way to do this is with biofeedback. Biofeedback teaches you how to control your body's response to stress. It involves using special equipment to measure your heart rate, skin temperature, and other vital signs. This information is then fed back to you so that you can learn to change your body's response to anger.

Meditation

Meditation is another great way to calm your anger. It involves focusing your attention on your breath and letting go of all other thoughts. This can be a very effective way to deal with stress and anger. You can become a neutral observer to your thoughts and emotions, without allowing them to consume you. Meditation practices that can help you master your anger are:

- **Transcendental meditation**. This is a popular form of meditation that uses a mantra to help you focus your attention.
- **Mindfulness meditation**. This type of meditation focuses on your thoughts, emotions, and sensations as they presently occur.
- **Guided meditation**. This is a type of meditation where you focus your attention on a particular object, such as a candle flame, your breath, or someone walking you through the meditation.

If you want to try meditation to calm your anger, be sure to start with smaller practices, focus on your breath to keep you grounded in the moment, and approach your anger from a different perspective.

Mindfulness

Mindfulness is a state of being aware of your thoughts and feelings without judgment (Holland, 2019). It can be very helpful in managing anger. When you're mindful, you can observe your thoughts and feelings without getting caught up in them. This allows you to see them for what they are and to let them go.

By being aware of your own heart rate and breathing and altering them as needed to reduce stress hormones, you can increase mood-enhancing hormones. Additionally, you'll decrease tension, irritation, stress, and anger; all of which are necessary to lead a healthy and productive life. It's important to remember that while these techniques can be helpful, they're not always easy. It takes practice to learn how to control your anger.

Chapter 9:

Anger Kills! Manage Your Anger

Anger is a powerful emotion that can have a big impact on your health. If you're not able to manage your anger, it can lead to several distinct health problems. These include high blood pressure, stroke, anxiety, heart disease, and depression.

By dealing with your anger efficiently, you'll avoid these health problems and live a healthier, happier life.

Responses to Anger

There are many ways that people respond to anger. Some people try to bottle it up, some lash out, and some just go completely blank. Figure out what works for your anger and the challenges you face.

Four Primary Ways of Expressing Aggression or Anger

There are four types of aggression: aggressive, passive-aggressive, passive, and assertive. Each type of aggression has its own set of characteristics. It's important to be aware of these so that you can identify when you're feeling angry and how to best express those feelings.

- **Aggressive**. Aggressive behavior is characterized by physical or verbal violence. This type of aggression is usually unplanned and can hurt feelings or even injuries. If you're feeling aggressive, it's important to find a constructive way to release that energy.
- **Passive aggressive**. Passive aggressive behavior is characterized by indirect expressions of anger. This can include sulking, procrastinating, or being critical. This type of aggression is often used to avoid conflict. However, it can still be harmful to relationships.
- **Passive**. Passive behavior is characterized by avoidance of conflict or confrontation. This can include ignoring the problem or walking away from the situation. Much like passive-aggressive behavior, this tactic is used to avoid confrontations. However, it can injure a relationship if the problem never gets resolved because of avoidance.
- **Assertive**. Assertive behavior is characterized by direct and honest communication. This type of aggression is usually the most effective in solving problems. It's essential to remain calm and respectful when using assertive communication.

How to Understand Your Anger

- **Recognize your anger**. The first step to managing your anger is to recognize when you're feeling it. Pay attention to your body and mind and try to identify the signs that you're getting angry. Don't try to bottle it down or ignore it. This will only make the situation worse. Accept that you're feeling anger and then focus on calming yourself down.

- **Identify your triggers**. If you can identify your triggers, you'll have an easier time controlling your anger. What are the things that make you angry? Once you pinpoint your triggers, you can avoid them or be prepared for them. This will help to prevent your anger from getting out of control.

- **Recognize the warning signs**. Before your anger gets out of control, there are usually warning signs. Pay attention to these signs so that you can take action before it's too late. These can include things like feeling tense, getting a headache, or feeling your heart rate increase. If you notice any of these signs, take a deep breath and try to calm down.

- **Pinpoint any negative self-talk**. One of the main things that can make anger worse is negative self-talk. This means that you talk to yourself in a way that makes you feel worse. For example, you might say things like "I'm so angry, I can't stand it" or "I'm never going to calm down."

This negative self-talk will only make your anger worse. Instead, try to focus on positive self-talk. This can include things like "I can handle this" or "I'm in control." This will remind you that you're in charge of your emotions and that you can handle the situation.

Emotion Regulation—DBT Skills

DBT skills can help you deal with your anger healthily. They can help you get in touch with your emotions, understand what is driving your anger, and develop a plan for responding to it constructively. The first step is to get in touch with your emotions. This means learning to recognize when you're feeling angry and to understand what is causing that anger. Then you can apply emotion regulation skills to improve your mood. Emotion regulation is a skill that helps you to change the way you respond to your emotions.

Changing the Way You Respond to Your Anger

Once you have a handle on your emotions, you can change the way you respond to them. This means finding healthy ways to express your anger instead of lashing out or bottling it up. Managing your anger might seem like an impossible task in today's demanding world. However, there are a few acronyms the DBT skills provide to assist with anger management. One of them is ABC PLEASE, which stands for **accumulate** positive experiences, **build** mastery, **cope** ahead, treat **physical** illnesses, **eating** habits, **avoid** mood-altering substances, maintain good **sleep**, and **exercise** regularly (Linehan, n.d.-a).

- **Accumulate positive experiences**. Think of your mind and body as a bank for a moment. You can make regular deposits of positive experiences into it, such as relaxation, vacations, fun activities with friends and family, etc. These act as a buffer against future stressors. Building up your "positive experience account" will help you have the emotional resources to deal with difficult situations when they arise.

- **Build mastery**. One way to manage anger is to have a sense of mastery over your life. This means feeling like you're in control of your life and that you can handle whatever challenges come your way. You can build mastery by setting goals and working towards them, learning new skills, and taking on challenging tasks. Hobbies are a great way to build mastery and still enjoy what you're working on.

- **Cope ahead**. This means planning for how you'll deal with difficult situations before they happen. This can help to prevent you from getting overwhelmed by your emotions and reacting in a destructive way. For example, if you know you're going to be in a situation that is likely to make you angry, plan ahead of time how you'll deal with it. This might involve practicing some relaxation techniques or coming up with a list of things you can do to calm yourself down.

- **Treat physical illnesses**. If you're dealing with a physical illness, it's important to get treatment for it. This will help to reduce the amount of stress in your life and make it easier to manage your anger. Our physical health can influence our mental health, so if you're concerned about your physical health, please see a doctor.

- **Eating habits**. What we eat can have a big impact on our mood and energy levels. Eating a healthy diet can help to improve our mood and give us the energy we need to deal with challenging situations.

- **Avoid mood-altering substances**. Substances like alcohol and drugs can make it more difficult to deal with our emotions. They can also make it more likely that we will act out in an aggressive or destructive way. If you're struggling with substance abuse, please get help from a qualified professional.

- **Maintain good sleep**. Getting enough sleep is important for our physical and mental health. When we're tired, we're more likely to get angry and react destructively. Try to get 7–8 hours of sleep each night.

- **Exercise regularly**. Exercise is a great way to release some pent-up aggression and keep your body healthy. It can also promote a positive mood and give us more energy to deal with difficult situations.

Ways to Handle Your Anger

There are many ways that you can handle your anger. To get the most out of your techniques, it's crucial to determine the best tips that work for your situation and to practice using those techniques when you're feeling angry. Some people find they need to use multiple techniques in order to effectively calm down.

- **Communicate your feelings**. It's important to communicate your feelings, especially when you're feeling angry. This will help to prevent arguments and hurt feelings. Try to share your emotions when you're calm so that you can have a productive discussion.

- **Exercise**. This can be a great way to release pent-up anger. Go for a run, lift weights, or take part in another activity that you enjoy. This will help to improve your mood and make you feel better, while also expelling the negative energy building inside of you.

- **Get some fresh air**. Going outside in nature is a great way to calm down and take a breather. Take a few deep breaths of the fresh, crisp air and focus on your surroundings, like the trees or blooming flowers. This will help to clear your head and make you feel more relaxed.

- **Use positive self-talk**. Once you've acknowledged your anger, start using positive self-talk to calm yourself down. This can include saying things like "I am capable of accomplishing this," or "I control the way I feel."

- **Distract yourself**. If you're feeling overwhelmed by anger, try to distract yourself. This can include watching a movie, reading a book, or listening to music. Doing something that you enjoy will distract your mind and make you feel more relaxed.

- **Practice relaxation techniques**. There are many relaxation techniques that you can use to calm yourself down. This can include things like deep breathing, progressive muscle relaxation, or visualization. Find a method that works for you and practice it when you're feeling angry.

- **Drop it**. Sometimes the best way to handle a situation is to drop it. This means that you let go of your anger and move on. Forgive the person or situation that made you angry—no matter how difficult it is. It will help you let go of your anger and focus on the positives in your life. Walk away and forget about it.

- **Improve your communication skills**. One way to improve your relationship with anger is to hone your communication skills. This means that you learn how to express yourself in a way that is respectful and doesn't hurt others. Be assertive, but not aggressive.

- **Set boundaries**. Another good way to deal with anger is to set boundaries. This means that you identify the things that make you angry and then set limits on them. For example, if you're getting angry because your boss is always yelling at you, you can set a boundary by telling them you won't tolerate being treated that way. This will help to protect you from getting angry in the future.

- **Practice empathy**. To better control your anger, you can practice empathy. This means that you try to comprehend how the other person feels. It's important to see things from their viewpoint. This will help you see the situation in a different light and possibly find a resolution.

- **Improve your problem-solving skills**. By improving your problem-solving skills, you can better manage your anger. This means that you learn how to effectively solve problems. It's important to find a solution that is fair to everyone involved. Hopefully, this will help to resolve the current problem and prevent future ones. Maybe you can be more open to negotiations or brainstorming solutions with the person who made you angry in the first place.

- **Practice makes perfect**. Remember that it takes time and practice to learn how to deal with anger. It's important to be patient with yourself and to keep trying. Eventually, you'll find the techniques that work best for you. Until then, just keep trying and don't give up. These abilities can eventually become a part of your normal behavior with enough practice.

- **Consider how to avoid the situation in the future**. After you've calmed down, think about how you can avoid the situation that made you angry. This will help to prevent the same situation from happening again and making you angry in the future. Maybe you can set boundaries or communicate more effectively.

10 "Quick Fixes" for Anger Management

1. **Take a few deep breaths**. Inhale slowly and deeply through your nose. Exhale slowly through your mouth. Repeat this for a few minutes.

2. **Visualize a peaceful place**. Close your eyes and imagine yourself in a calm and relaxing setting. It can be anywhere you want, such as a beach, a forest, or even your own backyard.

3. **Mantra and affirmations**. Choose a mantra or affirmation that you can repeat to yourself when you're feeling angry. This can be something as simple as "I am calm and in control." Repeating

your mantra or affirmation will help to refocus your thoughts and calm your mind.

4. **Do some muscle relaxation exercises**. Start by tensing and relaxing your toes, then work your way up to your calves, thighs, stomach, arms, neck, and face.

5. **Try box breathing**. This is a simple but effective relaxation technique that can help to calm your mind and body. Breathe in for a count of four, hold your breath for a count of four, breathe out for a count of four, and then repeat (Gotter, 2017).

6. **Alter your body's state**. Take regular cold showers or cold/ice baths. If you're new to cold therapy, start by applying a cold, damp cloth to your forehead or the back of your neck and then build up to putting your feet or hands in cold or iced water. Then you can move up to a cold shower and an ice bath immersion. By consciously putting your body in a controlled stressful situation, you're essentially practicing for real-life stressful situations. After a few seconds in the cold, your body learns to cope. As you breathe and focus, your mind and body relax and stress decreases. This response can be mirrored in your everyday life, so when stress is triggered, your mind and body are better equipped to deal with it. You could also hold your breath for 30 seconds to activate the brain's "dive" response, which can slow your heartbeat and make you feel more at peace. Changing the state of your body can help to change your state of mind.

7. **Opposite action**. Use the "opposite action" technique. This technique is a popular DBT exercise that prompts you to do the opposite of what your anger is telling you to do. For example, if your anger is telling you to scream, then you would try to stay calm and quiet. If your anger is telling you to hit something, then you would try to walk away or do something constructive.

8. **Use the acronym STOP**.

   - **S—Stop what you're doing**. This is the first and most important step. Once you're feeling angry, it's important to stop whatever you're doing. This will help to prevent the situation from escalating.

   - **T—Take a step back**. Once you've stopped what you're doing, take a step back from the situation. This will help to give you some distance and perspective.

   - **O—Observe what's going on**. Once you've taken a step back, observe what's going on around you. What triggered your anger? What are the facts of the situation? What are your thoughts and feelings?

   - **P—Proceed mindfully**. Once you've observed the situation, you can proceed mindfully. This means that you'll decide how to proceed in a deliberate and mindful way. You'll consider your options and choose the best course of action (Linehan, n.d.-b).

9. **4-7-8 breathing**. This breathing technique can help to calm you when you're feeling angry. Breathe in for four counts, hold your breath for seven counts, and breathe out for eight counts. Repeat this until you feel calmer.

10. **Let go of your anger**. After you've expressed your anger, it's important to let it go. This can be difficult, but it's necessary in order to move on. Try to forgive the person or situation that triggered you and focus on the joyous aspects of life. This will help you release your anger and progress.

Other Anger Management Tools

- **Take a timeout**. Timeouts aren't only for children! If you're feeling angry, take a few minutes for yourself to calm down. This can be a time to breathe deeply, relax, and think about what's going on.

- **Express your anger in a healthy way**. You don't want to bottle or hide your anger. Instead, release it in a healthy and creative manner. This can include writing, talking to someone, or physical activity. When you're able to speak clearly, be forceful yet non-aggressive when you vent your dissatisfaction.

- **Think before you speak**. It's easy to say things you'll later regret when you're angry. Before you say anything, take a few deep breaths and count to 10. This will help you calm down and think about what you're going to say.

- **Identify workable solutions**. When you're feeling angry, it's helpful to brainstorm potential solutions to the problem. This will help you feel more in control and less frustrated. Work on fixing the problem at hand rather than dwelling on the thing that enraged you.
- **Visualize peace.** Visualization is a powerful tool that can help you calm down. Close your eyes and imagine yourself in a peaceful, calm place. This can be anywhere that makes you feel happy and relaxed.
- **Use "I" statements**. When you're communicating with someone, use "I" statements. For example, instead of saying "You're so lazy!," try "I'm feeling frustrated because I need help with the dishes." This will help to avoid arguments and defensiveness.
- **Listen to music**. Listening to calming music can help to soothe you when you're feeling angry. Classical music is a great option, but any type of music that makes you feel calm and relaxed will work.
- **Write it out**. Writing is a useful and creative way to deal with anger. Write down your thoughts and feelings, or brainstorm potential solutions to the problem. This will help release stress and think more clearly.
- **Practice forgiveness.** Anger can be harmful to your health. It's important to learn to forgive both others and yourself. Forgiveness is a powerful instrument. You risk being overcome by your own resentment or sense of unfairness if you let anger and other negative emotions overpower the happy ones. This doesn't mean

that you forget about what happened or that you're condoning it. It just means that you're choosing to move on and let go of the anger and resentment.

- **Laugh.** Laughter can help reduce tension. It's a natural way to distract yourself from anger and focus on something positive. However, refrain from using sarcasm, since it might irritate others and worsen the situation. Watch a comedy film or funny TV show. Listen to a podcast that makes you laugh or go watch your favorite comedian.

- **Practice relaxation skills.** Relaxation techniques such as yoga, meditation, and progressive muscle relaxation can help you relax. Use your relaxation techniques when your anger flares. Develop your deep breathing techniques, visualize a soothing location, or mentally repeat a word or phrase that is comforting, such as "Take it easy."

Coping With Stress

Coping with stress is a lifelong journey. It's important to find what works for you and to be patient with yourself. Be gentle with yourself and keep trying different things until you find what helps you cope healthily. Remember, don't be afraid to experiment to figure out your best coping mechanisms.

Re-Balance Work and Home Life

A popular way to reduce stress is to find a healthy balance between work and home life. When you're able to focus on your relationships and hobbies outside of work, you're more likely to feel fulfilled and less stressed. Schedule time for your personal life and stick to it. This can be tough, but it's worth it.

Build in Regular Exercise

Exercise is a great way to reduce stress. Not only does it release endorphins, but it also gives you time to clear your head and focus on something other than your stressors. Try to exercise for at least 30 minutes a day, three times a week. This can be anything from going for a walk to playing tennis.

Eat Well and Limit Alcohol and Stimulants

Eating a healthy diet can help reduce stress. Eat plenty of fruits, vegetables, and whole grains. You should also limit your alcohol intake and avoid stimulants, such as caffeine and nicotine. Both can make stress worse.

Make Time for Relaxation

Relaxation is crucial for managing stress. Schedule some time each day to do something you enjoy, such as reading, listening to music, or spending time with friends and family. This can help you unwind and de-stress.

Connect With Supportive People

Social support is essential for coping with stress. When you have people you can rely on, it's easier to deal with stressful situations. Spend time with friends and family, and join a support group if you're dealing with a chronic stressor, such as illness or job loss.

Get Plenty of Sleep

Sleep is crucial for managing stress. When you're well-rested, you're better able to cope with stressful situations. Aim for seven to eight hours of sleep each night.

Practice Meditation, Stress Reduction, or Yoga

Meditation, stress reduction, and yoga are all great ways to reduce stress. These practices can help you focus on the present moment and let go of stressors.

Bond With Your Pet

Pets can be a significant source of comfort and support. If you have a pet, spend some time each day playing with or cuddling with them. Try grooming its hair or going for a walk. This can help reduce your stress levels and enhance your mood.

Take a Vacation

Vacations can be a great way to reduce stress. When you're able to get away from your everyday life, it's easier to relax and de-stress. Take a vacation at least once a year and go somewhere you've always wanted to visit.

Make Some Lifestyle Changes

If you're dealing with chronic stress, you may need to make some lifestyle changes. This can include things like simplifying your life, changing your diet, and getting more exercise. These changes can be tough, but they're often necessary to reduce stress in the long term.

See a Counselor, Coach, or Therapist

If you're struggling to cope with stress, it may be helpful to see a counselor, coach, or therapist. These professionals can help you identify the source of your stress and find healthy ways to cope.

Chapter 10:

Improve Your Social and

Interpersonal Skills

The social circle skill is the ability to effectively manage relationships with others. This includes being able to communicate effectively, set boundaries, and resolve conflict. When our social circle is healthy, we feel supported and connected to others.

We can have meaningful relationships that enrich our lives. When our social circle is unhealthy, we may feel isolated and alone. We may have difficulty communicating our needs or resolving conflict. Our relationships may be a source of stress instead of support. There are several things you can do to improve your social circle skills.

Interpersonal Effectiveness—DBT Skills

What Are Interpersonal Effectiveness Skills?

Interpersonal effectiveness skills are tips and practices that you can use in order to improve your ability to interact with other people. They're designed to help you build better relationships, communicate more effectively, and assert yourself in a way that's respectful and effective.

Why Are Interpersonal Effectiveness Skills Important?

Interpersonal effectiveness skills are important because they're the foundation of all human interactions. If you want to be successful in any area of your life, it's essential that you develop strong interpersonal skills.

What Are Some Tips for Using Interpersonal Effectiveness Skills?

Here are a few tips for using interpersonal effectiveness skills:

- **Be clear about what you want**. To communicate effectively, be clear about what you want. When you're interacting with someone, make sure that you know what your goal is. This will help you be more effective in achieving it.
- **Be assertiv**e. Another important tip is to be assertive. This means being able to express your needs and wants in a way that's respectful and effective. Assertiveness isn't the same as aggressiveness.
- **Be aware of your body language**. Another important tip is to be aware of your body language. Your body language can communicate a lot about how you're feeling and what you want. Pay attention to how you sit or stand, your facial expressions, and how you gesture your body.

- **Listen**. The ability to listen effectively is an important aspect of effective communication. When engaging in a conversation, make sure that you're really listening to what they're saying. Pay attention to the way they project themselves, their body language, and the pitch or tone of their voice. Try to understand their point of view.

- **Responding**. The ability to respond is another important aspect of communication. Respond to what they're saying, by asking questions or reiterating what they said. Acknowledge their points and offer your own counterpoints when necessary.

- **Asking questions**. Another important aspect of communication is the ability to ask questions. This will help to ensure that you agree and that you understand what they're saying.

- **Be respectful**. The final tip is to be respectful. This means listening to what other people have to say and considering their points of view. It also means being open-minded and willing to compromise.

Be Aware of Your Body Language

With communication, most of us only focus on the words. This makes a certain amount of sense—when we speak with someone, we choose the words that we think will convey our meaning in all its depth. But words only make up 7% of communication—the rest comprises tone (38%) and body language (55%). So, if you're only focusing on the words, you're only getting a fraction of the message across.

Instead, start paying attention to your body language. When you're speaking with someone, pay attention to your posture, facial expressions, and body gestures. Are you making eye contact? Are you leaning in or pulling away? Are you crossing your arms or opening them up? These things can communicate just as much—if not more—than the words you're saying.

Your body language is a form of nonverbal communication. Your body language can sway how others perceive you and how they respond to you. It's important to be conscious of your body language and make sure that it's sending the message you want to send.

Elements of Body Language

Eye Contact

Eye contact is one of the most important elements of body language. It's a form of nonverbal communication that can communicate a lot of information. When you make eye contact with someone, you're telling them you're interested in what they have to say. You're also telling them you're confident and trustworthy.

Facial Expressions

Facial expressions are another important element of body language. These expressions communicate a wide range of emotions, from happiness and sadness to anger and fear. Be conscious of your appearance and make sure that it's conveying the message you want to send.

Gestures

Gestures are another form of nonverbal communication. They can emphasize a point, express an emotion, or create a rapport with someone. Pay attention to your own gestures and make sure that they're sending the message you want to send.

Posture

Your posture is another form of nonverbal communication. It can communicate a lot about your attitude and your state of mind. Pay attention to your own posture and make sure that it's conveying the message you want to send.

Interpersonal Space

Interpersonal space is the space between you and another person. Pay attention to your own personal space and the personal space of others. Personal space can vary from culture to culture, so be sure to take that into account when interacting with someone from a different culture.

Tone of Voice

Your tone of voice is another form of nonverbal communication. It can communicate a lot about your emotions and your state of mind. Pay attention to your own tone of voice and make sure that it's properly conveying your intentions.

Be an Active Listener

The ability to listen is crucial to effective communication. When you're having a conversation, make sure you're paying attention to what they're saying. Focus on their body and tone of voice to understand their message. Try to understand their point of view. The ability to listen also involves being able to respond appropriately.

When you're speaking with someone, make sure that your response applies to what they've just said. If you're not sure how to respond, ask a question or make a comment that shows that you're interested in what they're saying. Communication is a two-way street—it's just as important to listen as it is to speak. When you're communicating with someone, make sure that you're doing both.

Areas of Interpersonal Skills

Communication Skills

Communication skills are just one part of interpersonal skills. Interpersonal skills are the skills that you need to interact with other people. They include communication skills, but they also include other important skills, like decision-making or conflict resolution.

Interpersonal skills are important in all aspects of life. They're especially important in the workplace, where you'll need to interact with co-workers, clients, and customers daily. If you want to be successful in the workplace, it's important to develop strong interpersonal skills.

Expressing your anger through productive outlets that don't hurt yourself or others is crucial. You could write or talk to someone or engage in physical activity. When you do feel angry, try to:

- **Share your emotions when you're calm**. When you're feeling angry, it's important to communicate your feelings. However, it's best to wait until you've calmed down before having a discussion. This will help to avoid arguments, hurting someone's feelings, or saying something you'll regret.
- **Avoid blaming**. When you're angry, it's easy to place blame. It was someone else's fault, or they should have known better. However, this will only make the situation worse. Instead of

blaming someone else, try to take responsibility for your own emotions and actions. Maybe there was something you could have done differently.

- **Assertiveness**. One way to handle your anger is to practice assertiveness. This means that you express your emotions healthily and stand up for yourself. It's important to avoid aggression and be assertive instead. This means that you should express your anger appropriately while being considerate of the other person.

Managing Differences

One of the most important aspects of interpersonal skills is the ability to manage differences. When you're interacting with someone, it's inevitable that you'll have some disagreements. It's important to manage those disagreements in a constructive way. Differences can arise for a variety of reasons, including:

- different values and beliefs
- different goals and objectives
- different ways of doing things
- distinct personalities

When you face a disagreement, it's important to remember that the other person isn't wrong—they just have a different perspective. It's also important to remember that you don't have to agree with everything that the other person says. However, it's important to be respectful of their opinions and their point of view. You can manage differences by:

- **Compromise**. Try to find the sweet spot that will make both parties satisfied and willing to agree on. This may involve making some concessions, but it's often worth it to reach an agreement.

- **Collaboration**. When you can't agree, try to work with the other person to find a solution that everyone can agree on. This may involve brainstorming ideas or coming up with a plan of action

- **Competition**. When you have a disagreement, try to win or to get what you want. This may involve trying to out-argue the other person or trying to get them to agree with your point of view.

Create a Harmonious Team

In order to be successful, it's important to create a harmonious team. A harmonious team is a group of people, like-minded or not, who collaborate together effectively. They have a common goal and they're able to cooperate with each other in order to achieve that goal. In order to create a harmonious team, there are a few things that you need to do:

- **Create a common goal**. The first step is to create a common goal. This is a goal that everyone on the team can agree on and work towards.

- **Develop a plan of action**. The next step is to develop a plan of action. This is a plan that outlines how you're going to achieve your common goal.

- **Assign roles and responsibilities**. The next step is to assign roles and responsibilities. This ensures that everyone on the team knows what their role is and what they're responsible for.

- **Communicate**. The ultimate step is to communicate. This ensures that everyone on the team agrees and knows what's going on.

Personal Integrity

Personal integrity is another important aspect of interpersonal skills. Personal integrity is the quality of being honest and trustworthy. It's about having a set of moral principles that you live by and being true to yourself. Personal integrity is important because it's the foundation of trust. Trust is essential in any relationship, whether it's personal or professional. If you want to develop personal integrity, there are a few things that you can do:

- **Be honest**. The first step is to be honest. This means being honest with yourself and with others. It also means being truthful and transparent.
- **Be reliable.** The next step is to be reliable. This means being someone who people can count on. It means keeping your word and following through on your commitments.
- **Be respectful**. The last step is to be respectful. This means treating others with respect and dignity. It also means being considerate of their feelings and opinions.

GIVE Acronym

The GIVE acronym is a tool you can use to enhance your interpersonal effectiveness skills. It stands for:

- **Gentle**. Be respectful and considerate in the way you speak to others.
- **Interesting**. Make sure that you're interested in what the other person is saying. Focus on their inflections, body language, and tone of voice.
- **Validate**. Acknowledge the other person's feelings and perspectives.
- **Easygoing**. Be flexible and open-minded in your interactions with others (Sunrisertc, 2017a).

FAST Acronym

The FAST acronym is another tool that you can use to improve your interpersonal effectiveness skills. It stands for:

- **Fair**. Be fair and just in your interactions with others.
- **Apologies**. Don't over-apologize. Only apologize when you've actually done something wrong.
- **Stick to your values**. Make sure that you're staying true to your own values and beliefs.
- **Truthful**. Be honest in your interactions with others (Sunrisertc, 2017a).

THINK Acronym

You can also use the THINK acronym to improve your interpersonal effectiveness skills.

It stands for:

- **Think**. Take a moment to think about the situation and the other person. Are they frustrated or angry too? Do the both of you think the other is unreasonable?
- **Have empathy**. Try to see the situation from the other person's perspective. What are they going through? How might they be feeling?
- **Interpretations**. Try to determine why the other person is acting the way they are. What are they hoping to gain or achieve? It helps to think about the most outlandish example first and whittle your way down to a more realistic interpretation. For example, if your partner is being short with you, instead of thinking "they must hate me," first think "they must be having a terrible day and they're taking it out on me."
- **Notice**. Pay attention to the other person's words, tone of voice, and body language. This will help you better understand how they're feeling. Maybe they smiled at you to show they understand how you feel.
- **Kind**. Respond to the other person in a kind and understanding way. You don't have to concur with their responses, but it does mean that you should try to understand where they're coming from (Sunrisertc, 2017a).

Boundary Building Skills

What Are Boundary Building Skills?

Boundary building skills are a set of techniques you can implement to improve your ability to set and maintain healthy boundaries. Boundaries are the limits that you set in order to protect yourself from being hurt, taken advantage of, or overwhelmed.

Why Are Boundary Building Skills Important?

Boundary-building skills are important because they help you create and maintain healthy relationships. When you have healthy boundaries, you're able to set limits in order to protect yourself. This allows you to have healthier relationships because you're not being taken advantage of or overwhelmed.

How Can I Improve My Boundary Building Skills?

There are a few key things that you can do in order to improve your boundary-building skills.

Learn the Boundaries

There are two types of boundaries: physical and emotional.

Physical boundaries are what you create to protect your body from pain, being abused, or becoming overwhelmed. Examples of physical boundary violations include:

- being touched without consent
- being forced to do something against your will
- having your personal space invaded

Emotional boundaries are the limits you instill to protect your emotions from being hurt, taken advantage of, or overwhelmed. Examples of emotional boundary violations include:

- being manipulated or controlled
- being gaslighted or subject to mind games
- being verbally abused or insulted

Understand the Boundaries

It's important to understand the difference between healthy and unhealthy boundaries. Healthy boundaries protect you, your body, and your emotions from being hurt or taken advantage of. Unhealthy boundaries are limits you set in order to control or manipulate others.

Some examples of healthy boundaries include:

- I won't tolerate being treated disrespectfully.
- I won't tolerate being taken advantage of.
- I won't tolerate being subjected to mind games.

Some examples of unhealthy boundaries include:

- I won't talk to you unless you apologize.
- I won't see you unless you meet my demands.
- I won't forgive you until you grovel and beg for forgiveness.

Identify Your Boundaries

The first step to setting boundaries is to identify what your boundaries are. This can be an arduous process, but it's important to take the time to really think about the limits that you want to set.

Some questions that you can ask yourself in order to identify your boundaries include:

- What are my deal breakers?
- What are my non-negotiables?
- What are my values?
- What do I need in order to feel safe, respected, and valued?

Communicate and Enforce Your Boundaries

Once you've identified your boundaries, it's important to communicate them to the people in your life. This can be a tough conversation to have, but it's important to be assertive and clear about what you're willing and not willing to tolerate.

It's also important to enforce your boundaries. This means that if someone violates them, you need to take action in order to protect yourself. This might mean ending a relationship, setting up new boundaries, or taking legal action.

Some examples of enforcing boundaries include:

- If someone doesn't respect your physical boundaries, you might need to end the relationship or take legal action.
- If someone doesn't respect your emotional boundaries, you might need to set up new boundaries or end the relationship.

- If someone doesn't respect your boundary of not being subjected to mind games, you might need to end the relationship.

Chapter 11:

Resilience and Resolution—

Building Strength

What Is Resilience?

Resilience is the ability to recover from or adjust easily to adversity or change. It's the ability to "bounce back" from tough experiences. Resilience is important because it helps us to cope with difficult situations and to recover from setbacks.

How Can I Build Resilience?

When you're struggling with anger, resilience can appear to be in short supply. However, you have the power to build resilience and to become more capable of managing your anger.

Some things that you can do to build resilience include:

- **Identifying your values and beliefs**. When you're aware and confident in your values and beliefs, you're more likely to hold firm in the face of adversity.

- **Building a support network**. A network of supportive people can provide you with emotional support when you need it.

- **Learning how to deal with stress**. Throughout this book, you've learned a wide variety of anger management skills. These skills can also help you deal with stress in a more constructive way. Putting these techniques into play in your day-to-day life will help you build resilience so you can manage your anger efficiently.

- **Identifying your triggers**. Awareness and understanding of your triggers are critical to managing your anger. When you know what sets you off, you can take steps to avoid or manage the trigger.

- **Developing a coping strategy**. You can't always avoid your anger, nor can you always change the situation that is causing your anger. In these cases, it's important to have a coping strategy in place. This might involve taking a time-out, journaling, or speaking to a friend.

- **Building emotional intelligence**. Emotional intelligence is the ability to be aware of and understand your emotions and the emotions of others. It's also about being able to regulate your emotions healthily. When you have emotional intelligence, you're more likely to respond to conflict constructively.

- **Practicing self-compassion**. You deserve to love and care for yourself just as you would for someone else. This includes being gentle with yourself, forgiving yourself, and accepting yourself. Sometimes, taking an hour or two for yourself can make all the difference in the world.

Building resilience takes time and effort, but it's worth it. When you have more resilience, you're better equipped to manage your anger and deal with conflict.

Developing a Growth Mindset

A growth mindset is a belief that your abilities and intelligence can be developed with effort and practice. This also applies to others and can be beneficial because it allows you to see conflict as an opportunity for learning and growth. When you have a growth mindset, you're more likely to:

- embrace challenges
- persevere in the face of setbacks
- learn from failures
- see mistakes as opportunities to grow

A growth mindset helps you in two ways. The first is by prompting you to understand that you have the ability to change. You're not stuck in the anger mindset, permanently set in your ways. You can learn new anger management skills and put them into practice. The second way is by teaching you that others can change. So, instead of getting angry when someone disappoints you, you can see it as an opportunity to help them learn and grow.

How to Develop a Growth Mindset

- **Acknowledge your strengths and weaknesses**. We all have areas we're good at and areas that we need to work on. Since you're reading this book, your anger is likely a weakness. What other weaknesses do you have? What strengths do you have? What is something you're irreversibly proud of yourself?

- **Be open to change**. If you're not open to changing your anger, then you won't be able to develop a growth mindset. You need to let go of your old anger management strategies and adopt new ones. The point of a growth mindset is that everybody is capable of change, so if you're not open-minded, then you can't change.

- **Be patient**. Change takes time. On average, it takes a person 66 days to develop a habit. So, if you're expecting to see results overnight, you're going to be disappointed. Be patient with yourself and trust that the process will work.

- **Be willing to put in the work**. A growth mindset doesn't happen overnight. It's something you have to work on every day. You need to put in the time and effort to develop a growth mindset.

- **Persevere in the face of setbacks**. You're going to have setbacks. That's inevitable. However, that's not the difference between failure and success. The difference is how you react to setbacks. Do you give up or do you keep going? If you want to develop a growth mindset, then you need to persevere in the face of setbacks.

- **Surround yourself with people who have a growth mindset**. If you surround yourself with negative people, then you're going to become negative. If you surround yourself with positive, growth-minded people, then you're more likely to adopt their mindset.

- **Embrace your mistakes**. Mistakes are inevitable. What matters is how you react to them. If you're able to learn from your mistakes, then they're not really mistakes. They're opportunities for growth. So, next time you make a mistake, don't beat yourself up. Embrace it and learn from it.

Six Steps to Build Resilience

Notice Your Stress Responses

In order to change your response to stress, you first need to be aware of your stress response. When you're feeling stressed, what do you do? Anger might be a significant stress response for you.

Some other stress responses include:
- withdrawing from others
- eating unhealthy food
- procrastinating
- sleeping too much or too little

- exercising less
- drinking alcohol
- isolating yourself

Once you're aware of your stress responses, you can change them.

Leave Your Mind and Turn to the Present Moment

When you're stressed, your mind is likely to wander. It might wander to the future and all the things that could go wrong, or it might wander to the past and dwell on things that have already gone wrong. You may continue to play out the argument or think about all the things you wished you would've said. This is normal, but it's not helpful. Take notes of when your mind is wandering and bring it back to the present moment. You can do this by focusing on your breath or by counting to 10.

Healthy Habits Are a Priority

When you're under stress, it's easy to let healthy habits fall by the wayside. You might skip meals, stop exercising, or start drinking alcohol to cope. However, these unhealthy coping mechanisms will only make you feel worse in the long run. It's important to prioritize healthy habits when you're under stress. Some healthy coping mechanisms include:

- eating a nutritious diet
- exercising regularly
- getting enough sleep
- connecting with friends and family
- taking breaks during the day

- practicing relaxation techniques

Find Meaning and Connect With Your Tasks

If you're feeling stressed at work, it's helpful to find meaning in your work. What is the purpose of your job? How does it help others? When you're able to connect with the meaning of your work, it can make the stress more manageable.

Empathy, Empathy, and More Empathy

Empathy for yourself. Empathy for others. Empathy for the situation. These things can help you manage stress. When you're upset or nervous, it's easy to be critical of yourself. You might think that you should be able to handle the stress or that you're not doing enough. Or, instead, you might blame others, claiming your reaction is their fault instead of your responsibility. However, these thoughts will only make you feel worse. Empathy can help you see the situation from all sides and understand that everyone is doing the best they can.

You Are the Driver of Your Life

You're in control of your life. You can't always control the circumstances, other people, or the outcome, but you can control your reaction. When you're overwhelmed, it's easy to feel like a victim. You might think that the stress is out of your control and that there's nothing you can do about it. However, this isn't true. The choice of how you react to stress lies in your hands. You can choose to let it consume you or you can choose to rise above it.

Remember, the anger or the situation isn't permanent. This too shall pass. No matter how bad the stress is, it's not permanent. It will eventually end. And when it does, you'll be stronger for having gone through it.

These are just a few tips to help you manage stress. Remember, you're not alone. We all deal with stress at times. And we can all cope with it.

Seven Cs of Resilience: A Formula for Success

When it comes to stress, we all face challenges. Life can be tough, and sometimes it feels like the weight of the world is on our shoulders. But we don't have to crumble under the pressure. We can build resilience— the ability to withstand difficult circumstances and even thrive despite them.

There's no one-size-fits-all approach to resilience. But there are some key ingredients that can help you weather any storm. These are known as the "seven Cs of resilience":

- **Confidence**. Trusting in your abilities and having faith in yourself.
- **Control**. Feeling like you can direct your own life and make choices that affect your future.
- **Commitment**. Sticking with your goals even when things get tough.

- **Challenge**. Embracing obstacles as opportunities for growth.
- **Change**. Accepting that change is a part of life and learning to adapt.
- **Coping**. Managing stress in healthy ways and developing positive coping mechanisms.
- **Connection**. Feeling connected to others and having a support system.

When you have the seven Cs of resilience, you have the power to overcome any challenge. So build up your resilience and face stress with confidence!

Chapter 12:

Cultivating the Right Attitude and Creating an Action Plan

It's essential to cultivate the right attitude for stress. Stress can be seen as a challenge or an opportunity. It all depends on your outlook. If you see stress as a negative force in your life, it will be. But if you see it as a chance to grow and learn, then it can be a positive experience. No matter what your attitude is, it's important to have a plan of action for when stress strikes. This way, you can be prepared and know what to do to minimize the impact of stress.

How Attitude Can Reduce Your Stress Levels

It's all in your head. The way you think about stress can have a big impact on how it affects you. If you view stress as a negative, it will be. But if you see it as a positive opportunity, then it can be just that. When you have a positive attitude, you're more likely to see stress as a challenge instead of a threat. This can help you feel empowered and in control. And when you feel empowered, you're more likely to take action and find solutions. So, don't underestimate the power of attitude.

It can make all the difference in how you deal with stress.

Thoughts Are the Creator of Experience

It's essential to have a positive thought process about your experiences with stress. A positive outlook will help you see the challenges instead of the threats. With some practice, we can increase our internal sense of serenity without changing other aspects of our life. Your thoughts create the experience you have, so why not make them positive?

How to Reframe Your Thoughts

If you're overwhelmed, it's easy to get stuck in a negative thought loop. You start worrying about all the things that could go wrong and before you know it, you're in a full-blown panic. But, there's a way to break out of this negative thinking cycle. It's called reframing. Reframing is all about changing your perspective. When you reframe your thoughts, you look at things in a new, more positive light. For example, let's say you're worried about a big presentation you have to give.

A negative thought might be, "I'm going to mess this up and everyone will think I'm a failure." But if you reframe that thought, you might say to yourself, "This is my chance to shine and show everyone what I'm capable of." See how changing your perspective can change the way you feel? When you're stressed out, try to reframe your thoughts in a more positive light. It may not be easy at first, but with practice, it will get easier. And the more you do it, the more resilient you'll become.

Some things that may help you have a more positive outlook toward stress are:

- regularly practicing gratitude
- focusing on your positive qualities
- challenging negative thoughts
- spending time with positive people
- doing things you enjoy

Creative Ways to Keep a Positive Attitude

It's easy to forget how to keep a positive attitude when you're in a negative mindset. But there are creative ways to stay positive, even in the face of adversity. Here are a few ideas:

- Write down three things you're grateful for each day.
- Start a gratitude journal.
- Make a vision board of all the things you want to achieve.
- Meditate or do yoga to center yourself.
- Spend time in nature.
- Listen to uplifting music.
- Practice deep breathing.

- **Regular self-care**. Have a regular sleep schedule, a healthy diet structure, and exercise often.

- **Start every morning strong**. Make it a habit to wake up early and take some time for yourself before starting your day.

- **Avoid spreading gossip**. When you focus on the negative, you attract more negativity. So instead of complaining about someone or something, try to find the good in the situation.

- **Be solution-oriented**. When you're anxious, it's easy to get caught up in all the problems. But, if you shift your focus to finding solutions, it can make all the difference.

- **Take actual breaks**. When you're taking a break, make sure you're actually disconnecting from work. That means not checking your email or scrolling through social media.

- **Crack jokes**. Laughter really is the best medicine. When you laugh, even amid stress, it can help lighten the load.

- **Have something to look forward to after work**. Whether it's meeting up with friends for dinner or going to your favorite yoga class, having something to look forward to can help you.

- **Focus on the long term, not the short term**. It's easy to get caught up on what's demanding your attention right now. However, take a step back and view the entire scenario from all aspects. Consider how it would impact the long-term.

- **Find a mentor**. Sometimes, it helps to have someone to look up to who's been through what you're going through. Find a mentor at work or in your personal life who can offer guidance and support.

How to Get Rid of Stress

If you're feeling overwhelmed by stress, you can incorporate techniques to get rid of it. Here are a few ideas:

- **Be healthy**. To fight stress, you can focus on taking care of your body. Visit the doctor regularly, eat well, and exercise.

- **Your mind is a sponge**. When you're anxious or overwhelmed, your mind may feel like it's full of negative thoughts. But if you take a moment to step back and observe your thoughts, you'll notice that they're just thoughts, not facts. This can help you view the situation in a more positive light.

- **Visualize your success**. It may be helpful to visualize your success when you're bombarded by stressors. See yourself achieving your goals and crossing the finish line. This can help you stay motivated and focused on what's important.

- **Disconnect from technology**. It's important to disconnect from technology and take a break from social media, email, and the news. This can help you relax and recharge.

- **Indulge in the calming power of aromatherapy**. Aromatherapy is a natural way to reduce stress. Try diffusing lavender or chamomile essential oils to create a calming environment. If you don't have a diffuser or oils, you can use scented candles or wall plug-ins.

- **Clean and declutter**. When your space is cluttered, it can add to your stress levels. Take some time to declutter and organize your space. This can help you feel more in control and less overwhelmed.

- **Time management**. To reduce stress, manage your time more effectively. This means setting priorities, making a schedule, and sticking to it. This can help you feel more in control of your time and less stressed.

Creating Your Action Plan

Now that you know some things that can help to reduce stress, it's time to create an action plan.

Here are a few ideas to get you started:

1. Make a list of the things that are causing you stress. This can help you pinpoint where in your life needs attention.

2. Identify the things that you can do to reduce stress. This can help you to create an action plan. Throughout this book, we've gone through several methods you can use.

   - DEAR MAN
   - GIVE
   - FAST
   - THINK
   - mindfulness techniques
   - ABC PLEASE

3. Make a commitment to yourself to reduce stress. This means making time for self-care and taking action to reduce stress.

4. Make a schedule and stick to it. This can help you make time for self-care and reduce stress.

5. Take action. This means taking the first step to reducing stress. This could be as simple as taking a few deep breaths or going for a walk.

6. Evaluate your progress. This means checking in with yourself periodically to see how you're doing. This can help you identify what's working and what's not.

7. Adjust your plan as needed. This can help you ensure that you're taking the best possible action to reduce stress.

Action Plan Template

Below is an action template you can follow or use as inspiration when creating your own. Identify your triggers and include as many effective treatment plans you think will help you overcome your stressors.

Situation 1:

My stressors (triggers): Describe the situation and the feelings you're experiencing. What happened?

_____

_____

_____

_____

Type of anger (destructive, passive-aggressive, hostile, etc.): Describe the anger you feel and the consequences that can occur if you act on it.

_____

_____

_____

_____

Treatment plans or coping mechanisms: What can you do to handle the situation more effectively?

Plan 1:

Plan 2:

Plan 3:

Plan 4:

Plan 5:

Situation 2:

My stressors (triggers): Describe the situation and the feelings you're experiencing. What happened?

Type of anger (destructive, passive-aggressive, hostile, etc.): Describe the anger you feel and the consequences that can occur if you act on it.

Treatment plans or coping mechanisms: What can you do to handle the situation more effectively?

Plan 1:

Plan 2:

Plan 3:

Plan 4:

Plan 5:

_____

_____

_____

By following these steps, you can create a stress reduction action plan and live a more peaceful life. Remember, it's important to be gentle with yourself and take things one step at a time. Rome wasn't built in a day, and neither is a stress-free life. So, take your time, be patient, and have faith in yourself. You can do this!

Conclusion

If you're struggling with anger, know that you're not alone. Many people have trouble managing their anger and it can be a tough emotion to deal with. However, there are many resources and techniques that can help you manage it healthily. This book has provided you with some techniques, information, and resources from in-depth research of proven methods that will help you control your anger and your emotions.

Don't let anger control your life—take back control, so you can live a peaceful and happy life. Here's a brief reminder of what you've learned so far:

- Anger is a regular and normal experience everyone has.

- Anger isn't always bad—it can be a motivator or a warning sign.

- It's possible to experience various forms of anger, such as constructive, destructive, hostile, passive, fear-based, physiologically based, etc. It's important to identify which type(s) of anger is/are affecting you to determine the best route you should take, which could be any of the following.

    ○ writing about your anger or keeping a journal
    ○ exercising to release the pent-up energy

- practicing meditation and mindful techniques
- talking to a trusted friend or a professional counselor/therapist

The steps to identifying and managing your anger are to:

- **Identify your triggers**. What makes you angry?
- **Learn to cope**. What can you do to make your anger subside and how can you prevent it from escalating?
- **Create a plan**. Write down what you'll do the next time you feel anger rising so that you have a plan to follow.
- **Practice your action plan**. If you practice consistently, it will become second nature.
- **Stay mindful of your anger**. Continue to be aware of when your anger rises and work to control it.
- **Re-evaluate your progress**. Check-in with yourself often and change your action plan as needed.

Anger management takes practice, and it's important to be patient with yourself. Start with small steps and work your way up. Remember to be kind to yourself and to seek professional help if you need it. You now have an armory full of tools to manage your anger in a healthy way, so put them to use and take back control of your life! If you found this book helpful, please share your experiences and leave a review so that others can benefit from it as well!

References

American Psychological Association. (2005). *Controlling anger — Before it controls you.* https://www.apa.org/topics/anger/control

Anger management - Self-management techniques. (n.d.). SkillsYouNeed.com. https://www.skillsyouneed.com/ps/anger-management.html

Beard, C. (2018, June 20). *5 reasons you're struggling to find balance in life.* The Blissful Mind. https://theblissfulmind.com/balance-in-life/

Breines, J. (2014, March 11). *Are some social ties better than others?* Greater Good Magazine. https://greatergood.berkeley.edu/article/item/are_some_ties_better_than_others

CBT Professionals. (2013, December 14). *The 7 c's of resilience* https://cbtprofessionals.com.au/the-7-cs-of-resilience/

Climan, A. (2021, August 16). *How anger management improves your life.* Verywell Health. https://www.verywellhealth.com/anger-management-5194513

Common dialectical behavior therapy DBT acronyms. (2018, January 23). Delray Center for Healing. https://www.delraycenter.com/common-dialectical-behavior-therapy-acronyms/

D'Arcy, G. (2021, May 27). *Stress balance: Understanding and counter-balancing stress.* D'Arcy Wellness. https://www.darcywellness.com/articles/stress-balance-understanding-and-counter-balancing-stress

Eddins, R. (2020, October 7). *Emotional regulation skills to cope with difficult emotions: [7 skills to practice today].* Eddins Counseling Group. https://eddinscounseling.com/emotion-regulation-coping-skills/

Felman, A. (2018, December 19). *Controlling anger: Tips, treatments, and methods.* MedicalNewsToday. https://www.medicalnewstoday.com/articles/162035

Greene, P. (2020, June 3). *Your easy guide to DBT's TIPP skills (a.k.a. TIP skills).* Manhattan Center for Cognitive Behavioral Therapy. https://www.manhattancbt.com/archives/1452/dbt-tipp-skills/

Holland, K. (2019, January 29). *How to control anger: 25 tips to manage your anger and feel calmer.* Healthline. https://www.healthline.com/health/mental-health/how-to-control-anger#1

The Jed Foundation. (n.d.). *Understanding anger.* https://jedfoundation.org/resource/understanding-anger/

Juneja, P. (n.d.). *Triggers or signs of work-life imbalance.* ManagementStudyGuide.com. https://www.managementstudyguide.com/triggers-or-signs-of-work-life-imbalance.htm

Linehan, M. (n.d.-a). *ABC please skill*. DBT Tools. https://dbt.tools/emotional_regulation/abc-please.php

Linehan, M. (n.d.-b). *ACCEPTS skill*. DBT Tools. https://dbt.tools/distress_tolerance/accepts.php

Linehan, M. (n.d.-c). *Boundary building skill*. DBT Tools. https://dbt.tools/interpersonal_effectiveness/boundary-building.php

Linehan, M. (n.d.-d). *Emotional regulation skills*. DBT Tools. https://dbt.tools/emotional_regulation/index.php

Linehan, M. (n.d.-e). *FAST skill*. DBT Tools. https://dbt.tools/interpersonal_effectiveness/fast.php

Linehan, M. (n.d.-f). *GIVE skill*. DBT Tools. https://dbt.tools/interpersonal_effectiveness/give.php

Linehan, M. (n.d.-g). *IMPROVE skill*. DBT Tools. https://dbt.tools/distress_tolerance/improve.php

Linehan, M. (n.d.-h). *STOP skill*. DBT Tools. https://dbt.tools/emotional_regulation/stop.php

Maintaining social connection in a time of physical distance. (2020, May 27). Kaiser Permanente Institute for Health Policy. https://www.kpihp.org/blog/maintaining-social-connection-in-a-time-of-physical-distance-2/

Mayo Clinic. (2020, February 29). *Anger management: 10 tips to tame your temper.* https://www.mayoclinic.org/healthy-lifestyle/adult-health/in-depth/anger-management/art-20045434

Morin, A. (2021, July 30). *11 ways to calm yourself fast when you're really mad.* Verywell Mind. https://www.verywellmind.com/anger-management-strategies-4178870

NHS. (2021, February 3). *Get help with anger.* https://www.nhs.uk/mental-health/feelings-symptoms-behaviours/feelings-and-symptoms/anger/

Pathak, N. (2000). *Mental health and anger management.* WebMD. https://www.webmd.com/mental-health/anger-management

Smith, M. (2019, March 20). *Anger management.* HelpGuide. https://www.helpguide.org/articles/relationships-communication/anger-management.htm

Smith, M. (2021, August 20). *How to take control of stress.* WebMD. https://www.webmd.com/balance/guide/all-stressed-out

Steinbrecher, S. (2017, November 7). *6 ways to build resilience and handle tough conversations.* INC. https://www.inc.com/susan-steinbrecher/6-

ways-to-build-emotional-resilience-perform-under-pressure.html

Sunrisertc. (2017a, August 18). *DBT distress tolerance skills: Your 6-skill guide to navigate emotional crises.* Sunrise Residential Treatment Center. https://sunrisertc.com/interpersonal-effectiveness/

Sunrisertc. (2017b, October 31). *Take control of your emotions using these 5 skills.* Sunrise Residential Treatment Center. https://sunrisertc.com/dbt-emotion-regulation-skills/

Sutton, J. (2021, June 24). *Your anger management guide: Best techniques & exercises.* PositivePsychology.com. https://positivepsychology.com/anger-management-techniques/

UC Berkeley (n.d.). *Understanding anger.* https://uhs.berkeley.edu/sites/default/files/understanding_anger_0.pdf

Understanding the 10 types of anger. (n.d.). Montreal CBT Psychologist. https://www.montrealcbtpsychologist.com/blog/122622-do-you-recognize-the-10-types-of-anger_8

Villines, Z. (2020, October 20). *Balance problems: Symptoms, diagnosis, and treatment.* MedicalNewsToday. https://www.medicalnewstoday.com/articles/balance-problems

Made in the USA
Columbia, SC
27 May 2024

36253515R00085